INFECTION CONTROL

The Critical Need to Wash Your Dirty Hands

TERESA D. MABRY

Independence University
April 2018

PAGE PUBLISHING, INC.
Conneaut Lake, PA

First originally published by Page Publishing 2020

ISBN 978-1-64462-004-5 (pbk)
ISBN 978-1-6624-3867-7 (hc)
ISBN 978-1-64462-005-2 (digital)

Printed in the United States of America

INDEPENDENCE UNIVERSITY

As members of the Final Project Committee, we certify that we have read the document prepared

by
Teresa Mabry

Infection Control: Critical Need to Wash Your Dirty Hands

and recommend that it be accepted as fulfilling the final project Requirement for the Degree of Germs or Infections

Master of Healthcare Administration

<u>Dr. Doret Ledford</u>   Date: <u>04/08/2018</u>
Dr. Doret Ledford, Course Instructor/AD/FPA

<u>Dr. Carmen Herbel</u>   Date: <u>04/23/2018</u>
Dr. Carmen Herbel Spears RN DHA MSN BSN Dean of the School of Healthcare

ABSTRACT

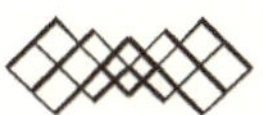

It is often a habit for people to go through the day without washing their hands. This is a constant throughout life, without them even thinking about the consequences of doing so. The dreadful number and related outcomes of those who do not wash their hands would probably shock many, especially those who eat out or encounter others throughout the day. Hence, the healthcare industry calls for bacteria control, or "infection control." Infection control refers to policies and procedures used to minimize the risk of spreading infections in both humans and animals, especially in hospitals or other healthcare organizations (Mosby's Medical Dictionary).

The policy of infection control aims to educate individuals on the importance of reducing the spread of infection. Pathogens are usually caused by bacteria or viruses, and can be spread by human–human contact, animal–human contact, and/or human contact with an infected surface. The diseases that spread from animals to humans are known as zoonoses; animals that carry disease agents from one host to another are known as vectors; thus, any person, people, or animals that transmit disease and place lives in danger for illness and even death. These issues that have been a concern since ancient times are critical even today. The subject has developed much research to include the most important corpus for reducing cross-contamination. Hence, investigators have examined the spread of infections and identified that the lack of handwashing is the primary reason for transmission of infections.

Keywords: Bacteria, infection control, transmission, cross contamination

CONTENTS

ACKNOWLEDGMENT

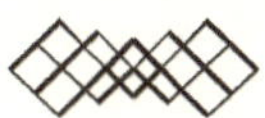

It is so inspiring to complete this fantastic journey; words cannot express it. Sometimes we think the road or walk is lonely, but when we allow the Heavenly Father to lead the way, he brings us to the destination—his way. I give Him the honor and the glory for giving me the opportunity to come to this place in my life where I was able to bring the desire to write a book into full fruition. I would like to thank my wonderful husband of thirty-eight years and my family's support, which is my backbone, and of course, we are thankful for our spiritual families who prayed.

We must not forget our educators, whom God placed in our lives to lead and guide us through this adventure. Dr. Ledford, I am so grateful for all your hard work, time, support, empathic listening, and encouragement to bring this thesis to completion. Hence, your words, in the beginning, were "we don't accept failure." Indeed, I had heard those words before, when a friend was praying for me during the path through respiratory school, and now, those same words have gotten me to the finish line once again. Thank you.

Emily Nevitt, I do not intend for you to go unmentioned; you definitely come to mind. All the beautiful emails and calls that you sent and made were during times when the path was dark. I could not see the finish line, but evidently, you did, so you kept sending, even when there was no answer until days or weeks later. Thank you, Emily, for the emails that made me smile and laugh. Thank you, Emily, for the stand you took to help me obtain back payment of my financial aid. Thank you, Emily Nevitt, I really appreciate your compassion and hands that continued to reach out to me. Emily, I am so grateful you were placed in my path on this adventure. Indeed, there are many instructors and individuals that I am grateful to but are not listed, like Monica Hartman and others who helped early in my journey, when I first enrolled at Independence University. I want to thank you!

CHAPTER 1

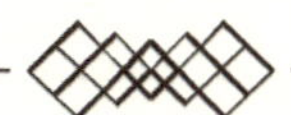

Introduction

Introduction to the Study

The statistics are dreadful, and even shocking, on the reasons why many become possessed with sickness and disease, and even face death, due to the lack of handwashing leading to cross-contamination with a germ of some sort. In 2012, statistics published by the Centers for Disease Control and Prevention (CDC) indicated that millions of Americans are affected by infectious illness annually (CDC 2012b). The CDC states that many communicable diseases can and should be prevented through measures such as vaccination and good health habits; however, proper handwashing is one of the most vital practices that protects oneself and others against communicable diseases (CDC, 2012). In 2015, the CDC stated that approximately 1 in 25 hospital patients had at least one healthcare-associated infection, which reflects the lack of hand hygiene and can result in the spread of germs in no time.

Cross-contamination is not limited to the healthcare industry; there must be awareness concerning this fact, especially for those who prepare food, since contact with any outside object while preparing food can transmit bacteria. People who eat out should also be alert to this issue because, although the United States' food supply is among the world's safest, they are also targets for cross-contamination.

A total of 9,000 Americans die each year as a result of food-borne illness, while millions are sickened due to the lack of education concerning the spread of disease (Hingley 1997). Although significant progress has been made in preventing the spread of infections, there is still much more work that needs to be done (CDC 2016).

It is essential to determine what is important when discussing cross-contamination or infection control, since the spread of disease must be eradicated. Thus, this subject is critical for dialogue, education, and reinforcement to prevent sickness or death. The proliferation of illness is a serious problem; For this reason, we will focus our attention on handwashing, which is a critical step that must be taken to control the spread of infections leading to illness or death (CDC 2016).

Several studies have indicated that the lack of handwashing contributes to individuals spreading staphylococcus, salmonella, clostridium, campylobacter, *Escherichia coli*, shigella, and *jejuni*. Transmission of disease thus occurs because one individual encounters a host and does not take time to wash his or her hands, thereby causing the germs to become prevalent. Cross-contamination is distance of one's involvement or understanding until contamination of a contagious infection hits home, leading to disease or even death. Therefore, handwashing underlies the fundamental principles and practices for preventing, controlling, and reducing the spread of infections and death (CDC 2016).

Recent disease outbreaks have justified that handwashing is one of most essential tasks persons can strive for throughout daily life. The outbreak of COVID-19 rapidly spread nationwide, claiming 1,035,341 lives in addition to 35,109,317 confirmed cases of COVID-19 including the president of the United States, Donald J. Trump and other officials in 2020 (WHO 2020). The outbreak has been critical for everyone to be educated on handwashing, hand sanitizer usage, and wearing of masks. The CDC (2020) announced recently the importance of washing hands because clean hands save lives. The organization said handwashing is not only simple and inexpensive, but can dramatically reduce the number of illnesses. The outbreak of COVID-19 is alarming for many, but the simple steps necessary to prevent such outbreaks are things like washing hands and educating others. It is an old practice that is taken for granted, but has brought about a critical alert for all of society.

CDC(2020)said handwashing education can:

Reduce the number of people who get sick with diarrhea by 23-40%, reduce absenteeism due to gastrointestinal illness in school children by 29-57%, reduce diarrheal illness in people with weakened immune systems by 58% and reduce respiratory illnesses, like colds, in the general population by 16-21%. Therefore, the COVID-19 pandemic provides a critical reminder to wash hands often and remember the common ways germs are spread (CDC 2020).

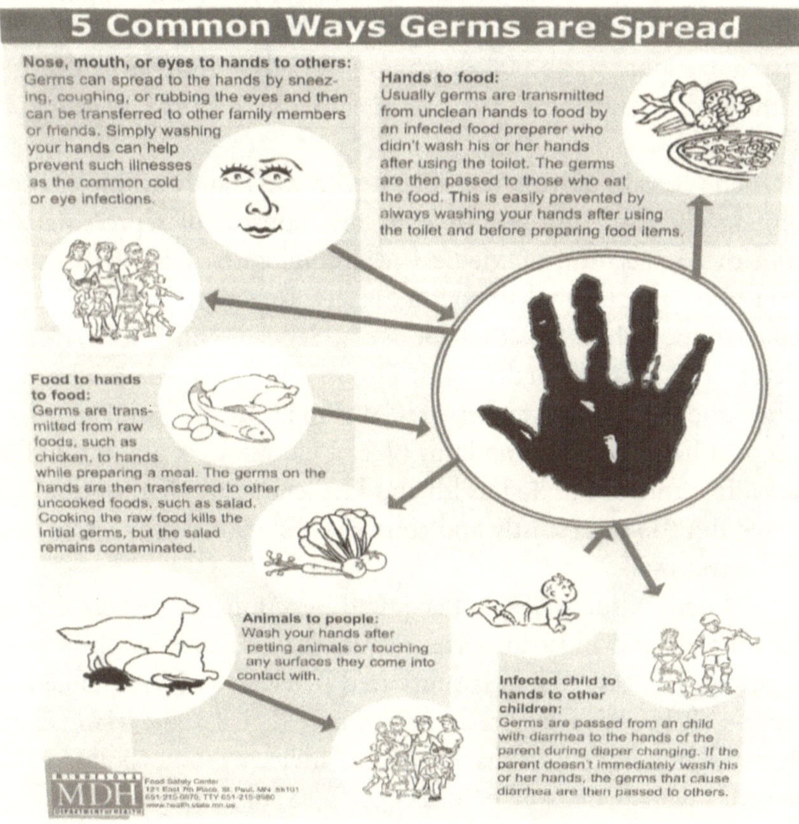

*Figure 1.1 5 Common ways germs are spread by Minnesota Department of Health.

The Global Public-Private Partnership for Handwashing(n.d.) states that washing one's hands with soap is a proven way to help prevent the spread of life-threatening diseases, especially among children. In fact, nearly two million children under the age of five die each year from diarrheal diseases and pneumonia. Moreover, there are many fighting the battle against cross-contamination. For instance, Dr.Harding, an associate professor at Oregon State University, FiDepartment of Public Health, acknowledges that as the purchase and consumption of meals from restaurants increases, proper and adequate hand hygiene at food preparation facilities is of increasing importance. Additionally, foodborne diseases have an impact on both public health and the economy at the local, national, and international levels. Approximately 76 million illnesses, 325,000 hospitalizations, and 5,000 deaths are caused by foodborne diseases in the United States annually (Mead et al. 1999; Pragle, Harding, et al. 2007).

The Royal Institute is affiliated with the Handwashing Liaison Group, which was formed in 1997 and consists of representatives from the Association of Medical Microbiologists, UK Department of Health, the Hospital Infection Society, Infection Control Nurses Association, Public Health Laboratory Service, and Public Health Medicine Environmental Health Group, and works to modify the behavior of healthcare workers (HCWs) to improve compliance with accepted handwashing standards (Teare, Cookson, et al. 2000). The Royal Institute of Public Health and Hygiene states that hospital-acquired infections are costly and consume vast amounts of scarce hospital resources.

Moreover, some hospital-acquired infections are preventable by the simplest and most important strategies that prevent the spread of germs. The easiest step is supported by clean and irrefutable evidence—all HCWs need to decontaminate their hands. Many clinicians and microbiologists have seen this advice be successfully implemented (Teare, Cookson, et al. 2000).

Background of the Problem

Infections have always been a significant cause of disability and death in humans worldwide. For centuries, little was known about what causes diseases or how to prevent or cure infections. By the 1800s, it was possible to identify some microorganisms that cause disease. For example, in 1846, a Hungarian doctor named Ignaz Semmelweis stopped thinking of illness as an imbalance created by bad air or evil spirits, and instead observed human anatomy. He collected data from patients on a maternity ward to research why so many women on the wards were dying, and he counted the number of deaths on each ward. Semmelweis noticed that there were particles, or small pieces of a corpse, on the hands of individuals who performed the autopsies, which were then transmitted to the women on the maternity ward due to the lack of handwashing. Semmelweis ordered his medical staff to start cleaning their hands and instruments. His proposal contributed to a dramatic decrease in the number of deaths (Davis 2015).

Moreover, with more advanced studies on the cause of infections and how to cure and prevent disease, the discovery of sulfa and penicillin in the 1930s encouraged the fight against infections. However, over the next six decades, antimicrobials have been developed to fight bacterial, fungal, and viral infections. It seemed the battle against infection was won, until the rapid and global spread of drug-resistant bacteria began to threaten the effectiveness of all currently available antimicrobials (Turkoski 2005). Then, a new phase of the war against infection began, and the search for methods to reduce the spread of this drug-resistant bacteria began (Turkoski 2005).

Therefore, it is essential to return to the basics of handwashing, since for more than a century, it has been a primary practice recommended to curtail the spread of infectious agents transmitted by human contact. Indeed, evidence of its effectiveness has recently been reviewed with a measurable positiveness that handwashing reduces infections (Larson, Early, et al. 2000). Further, briefly going back in time once again, we can note that even during frontier days, the value of disinfectants was recognized; a common practice was cleaning one's hands and instruments with whiskey (Lusk 1996).

Statement of the Problem

Society is full of widespread infections and diseases that have become resistant to antibiotics, because a majority of the time, people lack proper hand hygiene and cleanliness. People are often lax in washing their hands once a contaminated object or person has been touched. Hence, with a growing epidemic of new types of germs that mutate regularly, individuals tend to disregard the importance of handwashing and continue with their busy daily lives, ignoring the lack of habits and education necessary to engage in the critical need to stop and wash one's hands. Therefore, cross-contamination continues to be prevalent in our society, not only in the healthcare field but also in the community.

Thus, as hands carry many bacteria, and cross-contamination is possible without good hand hygiene; even shaking another person's hand who has not taken the initiative to wash can lead to illness. The hand carriage of resistant pathogens has repeatedly been shown to be associated with various types of infections, including nosocomial infections. Hands are commonly colonized with pathogens such as methicillin-resistant *S. aureus* (MRSA), *vancomycin-resistant Enterococcus* (VRE), *MDR-Gram-negative bacteria* (GNBS), *Candida Supp, Clostridium difficile*, and staphylococcus, which can survive for as long as 150 hours on the skin(Mathur 2011).

The resistance to or lack of discipline for hand hygiene creates serious problems, and even death, since the hands may become adulterated by merely touching a dirty object, person, money, or food, which will lead to the prevalence of germs if the person does not then wash his or her hands. It is critical for humans to wash daily, since approximately ten skin epithelial cells containing viable microorganisms are shed daily from healthy skin (Mathur 2011).

Purpose Statement

The purpose of this study was to educate individuals on the importance of handwashing and the health hazards that arise from not washing one's hands. "Anti-infectiousness is to wage war: to wage and win the war against a variety of infective organisms that cause so much human misery and death." Indeed, individuals must be educated about how diseases are spread. The chance of a person's hands encountering contaminated objects and surfaces is heightened in public places, such as educational institutions, restaurants, and hospitals. Thus, without a unified sense of responsibility to keep from coming in contact with and spreading illness-causing pathogens, health risk becomes a primary concern.

Successful programs designed to promote public health through the collective effort of community members rely on the careful evaluation of program effectiveness to bring about desired outcomes, including behavioral changes. Therefore, it is essential to investigate the efficacy of handwashing and related education (Burusnukul and Broz 2013).

Objective of the Study

This book has several unbiased and biased schemes, in order to expose some of the madness of individuals who do not wash their hands or fail to wash them correctly. Handwashing can be a challenge for HCWs and visitors because of the lack of education of the importance of washing hands to prevent cross contamination. Of course, some persons fail to wash their hands for various behavior rationales. Thus, this study's objectives are as follows:

- To assess the effect of an intervention to prevent the spread of infections, promote hand hygiene, and investigate risk factors for noncompliance with handwashing (Hugonnet, Perneger et al. 2002);

- to assess knowledge, attitudes, and practices toward the spreading of infections, and
- to evaluate the effects of handwashing on the reduction of healthcare- and environmental-associated diseases, as well as other types of cross-contamination (Madrazo 2009).

Research Questions and Hypotheses

Handwashing is vital to the health and welfare of everyone, but especially vulnerable populations in healthcare facilities. Therefore, the research questions are as follows:

1. Will handwashing hygiene prevent infections?
2. Are handwashing practices related to healthy behaviors?
3. Is hand-rubbing with an alcohol-based solution more efficient in reducing hand contamination than handwashing with soap and water?

The hypotheses created from these questions are as follows:

H1a: Those that utilize good hand hygiene contribute to the prevention of infections

H1o: Those that do not utilize good hand hygiene are less likely to prevent infections.

H2a: The practice of handwashing could be related to behaviors.

H2o: The practice of handwashing is not related to behaviors.

H3a: Hand-rubbing with alcohol-based solutions may be more effective in reducing contamination than washing with soap and water.

H3o: Hand-rubbing with alcohol-based solutions is not more efficient in reducing hand contamination than washing with soap and water.

Assumptions

Often, humans take things for granted, of which handwashing seems to be one. Hence, the decision to not wash one's hands will affect a person's health and the health of others around them, according to an article published by an unknown in *Teen Vogue(n.d)*. The publication usually is not the best source for resource data. However, many young persons read the magazine. The persons that do read the magazine is a generation that must be informed about cross contamination and how the lack of hand washing will transmit bacteria that could be deadly. The hands can be vectors that help transmit bacteria and viruses from one place to another, since people pick up bacteria and germs when the face, nose, mouth, and surfaces are touched.

If one's hands are washed, it interrupts the transmission of disease from one person to another or from all surfaces that are encountered. However, if one's hands are not washed, this transmission would not be interrupted, thus providing bacteria and viruses more opportunities to use one's hands as a way to move from one place to another and cause sickness and/or death (Vogue 2017).

Limitations of the Thesis Study

One of the limitations related to this study is the sole focus on handwashing to reduce the spread of infections. There are many areas that this study will not cover, because the subject of infection control is so broad and handwashing approaches and strategies are numerous. Another limitation is that the information for this thesis was extracted from several studies, which are secondary data; however, the material is critical to share. For example, in a study titled "An organizational climate intervention associated with increased handwashing and decreased nosocomial infection," the researcher posits that influencing habitual behaviors, such as handwashing is extremely difficult as there is resistance against it, especially in challenged healthcare settings (Larson, Early, et al. 2000). Healthcare setting are challenged in preventing cross-contamination because of education, and some persons or organizations not taking the spread of infections seriously.

Definitions of Terms

Bacteria are a domain of life existing as small, unicellular microorganisms. The genera vary morphologically, being spheric (cocci), rod-shaped (bacilli), spiral (spirochetes), or comma-shaped (vibrios). The nature, severity, and outcome of any infection caused by a bacterium are characteristic of that species (Medical Dictionary 2003–2013).

Cross-contamination is the transfer of infection directly from one person to another, or indirectly from one person to another via a fomite (Farlex, Medical Dictionary 2012).

Infection control refers to policies and procedures used to minimize the risk of spreading infections, especially in hospitals and human or animal healthcare facilities (Medical Dictionary 2003–2018).

Staphylococcus aureus are organisms found in humans and in the environment—in dust, air, sewage, and on the hands. The bacteria are spread primarily by food handlers using poor sanitary practices (Gale Encyclopedia 2006).

Summary

The shocking statistics regarding cross-contamination have generated some serious issues within our society; thus, they must be addressed to educate, inspect, and reinforce rules, signs, and laws when it comes to handwashing or practicing cleanliness. It takes discipline, or an infection, to hit home before persons take handwashing seriously. Handwashing is a fundamental principle and practice in the prevention, control, and reduction of acquired infections (Bjerke 2004).

CHAPTER 2

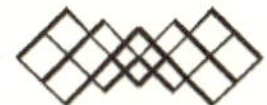

Literature Review

Overview

Though diseases have been a chief origin of impairments and death in humankind worldwide; it is time to take action by knowing the importance of speaking out about cross-contamination and educate people on understanding the origin of cross-contamination. Prior generations, knew little about the causes of infection, how to prevent or cure infection. With the discovery of penicillin in 1928 and sulfa in 1935, the ability to fight infection became a reality. Over the next six decades, antimicrobials were developed to fight bacterial, fungal, and viral infections. It seemed the battle against infection was won, until the rapid, global spread of drug resistant bacteria began to threaten the effectiveness of all currently available antimicrobials. Indeed, a new phase of the war against infection began, and the search for methods of reducing the spread of drug resistance began (Turkoski 2005). However, to win the war on cross-contamination, it would take informing those in healthcare and the public of how disease spreads. Handwashing can be a challenge for some healthcare personnel and visitors due to the lack of education on cross-contamination. Thus, making people aware of the importance of good hand hygiene and putting these actions in practice would be a simple step to prevent the spread of infections. These suggestions to prevent cross-contamination by practicing washing one's hands can and will

23

win the battle on infecting others with bacteria. Thus, this answer, in a broader sense, is infection control. Infection control is a term for preventing and stopping the spread of infections within the health-care setting (CDC 2016).

However, germs and bacteria are not retained in healthcare settings if individuals do not initiate the proper steps to prevent the spread of disease to the outside environment or a host. Handwashing is the simplest step for the prevention and inhibition of cross-contamination. A healthcare setting can contain many contagious infections that can spread to outside of the hospital and other persons or objects. Due to the emergence of numerous bacteria in the world today, it is interesting that the study of cross-contamination and human bacteria is prevalent in our era; although some bacteria are good for the human body and must remain intact. A study completed in 1972 by Luckey estimated that there are a total of 10^{13} bacteria in the human body. The study used a ratio of bacterial cells to human cells and said that there were $10^{(14)}/10^{(13)}$ bacterial cells in human cells. This means that there is a 1:10 ratio of bacterial cells to human cells (Sender, Fuchs and Milo 2016). Therefore, as various types of bacteria increase globally, it is no surprise that bacteria cells outnumber natural body cells; since the spread of infectiousness diseases continue to mutate. Thus, this is another critical reason why ongoing research is needed to prevent and stop the spread of infections, especially since it is taking higher doses of antibiotics to kill various bacteria. Mackenzie(2016) wrote many more people could die from common bacterial infections, as resistance to antibiotics booms and infections become untreatable.

Of course, previous research on the ratio of bacteria to human cells is not set in stone and was not intended to be the final word—especially since there was criticism from the start. However, Luckey, who studied the theory, posited that bacteria are found in many parts of the human body, primarily on the external and internal surfaces of the body, including the gastrointestinal tract, skin, saliva, oral mucosa, and conjunctiva. Indeed, the significant amounts of commensal bacteria that reside in the colon and the skin are vital to educate others so daily hygiene would be perpetual. The skin, although exposed to many bacteria, has protection to shield from infections; however, one could be infected by bacteria if there is a break in the skin, and/or one could be the host that starts a disease outbreak. Germs are a part of everyday life, are found in the air, soil, and water. Therefore, it is essential to wash one's hands and recognize three sources that the CDC (2016) says are necessary for an infection to occur:

- Place where infectious agents (germs) live (sink, surfaces, human skin, money)
- Susceptible person—a way for germs to enter the body
- Transmission—how bacteria are moved to a susceptible person.

Centers for Disease Control and Prevention

The CDC—an expert in the realm of infection control—identifies three sources of infections. They describe a source as an infectious agent or germ, which refers to viruses, bacteria, or other microbes that are found in many places, including on patients, HCWs, visitors, household members, and money. It is also true that people can be sick without symptoms of an infection or be colonized with germs, asymptomatic, but able to pass the germs to others. The other environmental sources where germs can be found or formed are as follows:

- Dry surfaces in patient care areas, public bathrooms and doorknobs
- Wet surfaces, moist environments such as cooling towers, faucets, and sinks
- Indwelling medical devices (catheters and IV lines)
- Dust or decaying debris, such as construction dust or wet materials from water leaks (CDC 2016)

Bacteria are easily transmitted, and some individuals are easily susceptible. For instance, in people that have not been vaccinated or those with weak immune systems, bacteria can enter the body and invade tissues, multiply, and cause a reaction (CDC 2016). Germs can have access to a person prone to infection by way of devices such as IV catheters or surgical incisions.

Furthermore, the CDC declares that healthy immune systems can help fight foreign invaders. However, the organization also cautions that, when a person's immune system is in some way compromised, or he/she is sick and needs to receive medical treatment in the hospital, there are some factors that can increase one's susceptibility to infections:

I. Patients in healthcare settings who have underlying medical conditions, such as diabetes, cancer, and organ transplantation, because of their reduced immunity(the body's inability to fight the infection)

II. Certain medications used to treat medical conditions, such as antibiotics, steroids, and certain cancer-fighting medications, increase the risk of some types of infections. Using antibiotics for viruses can put one at risk of getting a bacterial infection that is resistant to antibiotic treatment (Federal Drug Administration (FDA), 2019). Antibiotic resistance to antimicrobial agents was detected for the first time in the late 1950s and early 1960s (Aslam et el., 2018).

III. Life-serving medical treatments and procedures used in healthcare, such as urinary catheters, tubes, and surgery, because they provide ways for germs to enter the body.

Transmission is the third way the CDC states that infections occur. The organization says that bacteria must have a host, because germs do not maneuver themselves. The transmission of germs depends on people, the environment, and/or the type of equipment. Therefore, cleanliness is always essential, since germs travel through contact (touching), sprays, splashes, inhalation, and sharp injuries (individuals accidentally injected with used needles or hurt with sharp instruments). The CDC has tirelessly led the fight against disease; hence, the organization has published essential information to educate people and reinforce practice compliance to decrease cross-contamination. Certainly, these resources provide great insight for individuals to change their attitudes and behaviors when it comes to hand hygiene and the importance of ensuring germs are not directly or indirectly transmitted to others. Thus, the material published on transmission of infection includes the following:

I. Contact moves germs by touch (MRSA or VRE); for instance, hands of individuals who do not wash them can become contaminated by touching items that contain germs, and then germs are carried on the hands and spread to a susceptible person, if proper handwashing is not performed before contact is made.

II. Sprays and splashes occur when an infected person coughs or sneezes, creating droplets that carry germs over short distances (within approximately 6 feet). The microbe can land on a susceptible person's eyes, nose, or mouth and can cause infection (pertussis or meningitis).

III. Inhalation occurs when germs are aerosolized into tiny particles that can survive on air currents over great distances to reach a susceptible person. Thus, when germs are aerosolized by medical equipment or by dust from a construction zone (nontuberculous mycobacteria or Aspergillus).

IV. Injuries from sharps can lead to infections (HIV, HBV, and HCV) when blood-borne pathogens enter through a skin puncture, made with a needle or another sharp instrument (CDC 2017).

World Health Organization

The World Health Organization (WHO) was established in 1948, and is a specialized agency of the United Nations, serving as the directing and coordinating authority for international public health matters (Peden, et al, 2004). It is important to mention that an investigation implemented by WHO between 2000–2013 provides evidence that hand hygiene reduces transmission and infections by multi drug-resistant organisms (MDROs) in healthcare settings. The investigation will prove the importance of good hand hygiene. The review primarily focused on studies where hand hygiene was the key intervention implemented, and hand hygiene indicators (hand hygiene compliance and/or alcohol-based hand rub (ABHR) product consumption) were measured along with MDRO infection and/or transmission rates. The study found that infections caused by MDROs are increasing worldwide; therefore, it is critical and urgent to prevent the spread of MDROs, because the number of antibiotics available to treat these infections is extremely limited, and the development of new antibiotics is not forthcoming (WHO 2000–2017).

How much more straightforward can the message concerning the urgent need to prevent cross-contamination get? Hence, the WHO even mentions that the resistance in these microorganisms has mainly been caused by inappropriate use of antibiotics; however, contaminated hands, items/equipment, and environments often lead to outbreaks and serious infections. Therefore, implementing standard precautions for all and at all times is key to preventing the spread of all microorganisms, and MDROs in particular, noting that hand hygiene is the most important measure among standard precautions to prevent cross-contamination (WHO 2000–2017).

Cost

Some interesting information was published by WHO. Hence, reports on hand hygiene are reported to cost but show some benefits from the actions from washing hands. According to Chen and colleagues(2013), prominent investigators mentioned in WHO that every $1 spent on hand hygiene promotion could result in a $23.7 benefit. Similarly, Pittet et al(2004). reported that the total cost of hand hygiene promotion corresponded to less than 1% of the costs associated with nosocomial infections. In another study by Carboneau and colleagues, the overall prevention of 41 MRSA (Methicillin-resistant S Aureus) infections resulted in a gross savings of $354, 276, with a net hard dollar saving of $276,500. Moreover, according to a stochastic mathematical model, a 200-bed hospital incurs $1,779,283 annually in MRSA infection-related expenses attributable to hand hygiene noncompliance. In this setting, the model estimated that a 1% increase in hand hygiene compliance would result in annual savings of $39,650 (WHO 2013).

Behaviors

Researchers are paying more attention to habit formation and behaviors to improve compliance with handwashing. In 2000, a study was published by a team of researchers led by Elaine Larson. They first addressed the issue of how much handwashing is enough, and whether more frequent or better handwashing had an incremental impact on the reduction of risk of hospital-acquired infections. They concluded, "Even in this era of multiple precautions, several studies in the 1990s have demonstrated that staff handwashing led to a measurable positive effect on nosocomial infection rates" (Larson, et al., 2000). Larson continued to elaborate that "continued emphasis on hand care regimens seems justified, and if that is the case, another challenge of the handwashing behavior of healthcare professionals has proved to be stubbornly resistant to intervention and change" (Larson, et al., 2000).

Additionally, Larson further elaborated that everything from peer pressure to social mores can affect hand hygiene compliance. However, she found that supervisors and organizational culture can be more influential than expected. Thus, her 15 studies were designed to improve handwashing, gloving, and universal precaution practices among healthcare professionals, and interventions included various educational strategies, performance feedback, and environmental controls or modifications; however, only two of the studies reported any sustained behavioral effects on rates of infection (Pyrek 2004).

Over one year, multi-faceted interventions, including focus group sessions, installation of automated sinks, and feedback to staff on handwashing frequency—were implemented in an ICU. The variables observed were handwashing frequency, self-reported practices, and opinions about handwashing. During 301 hours of observation, 2,624 instances of handwashing were recorded. The proportion of times hands were washed varied by indication, ranging from 38% before invasive procedures to 86% for dirty to clean procedures ($p < 0.00001$). The researchers concluded that:

> Although there were some significant differences between the experimental and control units in handwashing during the study, these differences had returned to baseline by the two-month follow-up. There were no significant differences in self-reported practices and opinions from before to after intervention, nor between units. Thus, intensive intervention, including feedback, education, and increased sink automation, had minimal long-term effects on handwashing frequency. (Pyrek 2004)

Handwashing and Food Handling

Food handling is a significant issue when it comes to proper hygiene. Food handler focus groups in two counties in Oregon discussed their perspectives on handwashing behaviors and barriers in the restaurant environment. Factors that were suggested as barriers included food-handling practices, food handlers' perceptions, restaurant's kitchen policies, lack of supervisory or peer support, and lack of proper equipment such as sinks, hot water, and soap (Clayton et al. 2002; Dippold, Lee, Selman, et al. 2003; Green and Selman 2005; Howes, McEwen, et al. 1996). Thus, observational studies have found unacceptably low rates of hand hygiene practices (Clayton and Griffith 2004; FDA 2004; Green et al. 2006). Because barriers to handwashing are multidimensional in nature, a program that addresses factors identified by focus group participants is needed. This program might include the following:

- A hands-on training program to orient new employees to correct handwashing practices
- Involvement of both managers and coworkers in new employee handwashing training
- Emphasis on providing an attractive and clean sink for handwashing, equipped with necessary supplies
- Continued handwashing training and support involving the foodservice industry, managers, and coworkers
- Involvement of health departments and inspectors in providing managers and food workers with advice and consultations regarding the improvement of handwashing practice.

Indeed, researchers emphasize that it is essential that measures are taken to improve the Health Department and Healthcare inspectors' dialogue concerning good hand hygiene while handling food produces and ways to enhance handwashing interventions. The study demonstrated the effectiveness of research that seeks to include the experience and knowledge of food workers, currently working in the restaurant business, and showed that the qualitative approach of a focus group provides rich and detailed data about barriers that food workers perceive to handwashing. Thus, continued research with involvement from food workers should improve the effectiveness of these programs, as well as contribute to a broader understanding of effective handwashing strategies (Pragle, Harding, Mack 2007).

Drivers and Motivations for Handwashing

Burusnukul and Broz—the authors of a study completed at a university in the American Southwest—aimed to determine the efficacy of a four-year campaign implemented by the university's health services department. This campaign consisted of posting signs in lavatories across campus to remind students, faculty, and staff to wash their hands after using the facilities. This study provides evidence that the use of handwashing signs posted around common areas yields positive results (Arendt and Sneed 2008; Pragle et al. 2007). Researchers say signs or posters help to reactivate the information that individuals may already have received in previous sanitation education concerning handwashing (Allwood et al. 2004). Burusnukul and Broz indicated that not only are signs essential, but the availability and accessibility of handwashing facilities and supplies have been linked to influencing handwashing behavior in foodservice settings, where it is especially critical (Green et al. 2007). It is noted that hand-washing sinks available in multiple units significantly promote foodservice workers' handwashing behaviors. Conversely, limited numbers of sinks or sinks placed in inconvenient locations were consistently noted to hinder handwashing in focus group interviews (Green and Selman 2005). Thus, similar influences may be expected in the realm of public health practices. Indeed, by ensuring that handwashing supplies and equipment are always available and in working order encourages and enables individuals to wash their hands more frequently (Burusnukul and Pattarapong 2013; Pragle et al. 2007).

Moreover, this study focused on the students' and employees' predisposing characteristics (i.e., handwashing beliefs, attitudes, and knowledge) toward handwashing behaviors and the effect of hand-washing-reminder signs as an enabling factor. The investigation was twofold. First, the study assessed the following:

- Beliefs about handwashing
- Attitudes toward handwashing
- Knowledge of handwashing

Secondly, the study was to determine the effectiveness of the "Clean Hands Campaign" initiated university-wide, by assessing individuals' awareness of the investigation. Its awareness of the effectiveness of handwashing and how the program affected university students' and employees' engagement in adequate and proper handwashing behaviors (Turkoski 2005).

Normal Bacterial Skin Flora

Knowledge of normal bacterial skin flora is essential. Normal human skin is colonized with bacteria; different areas of the body have varied total aerobic bacterial counts (e.g., 1x 106calony forming units (CFUs)/cm2 on the scalp, 5×105(FUs/cm2in the axilla, 4×104 CFUs/cm2 on the abdomen, and 1x 104 CFUs/cm2 on the forearm). Total bacterial counts on the hands of medical personnel range from 3.9×104 to 4.6×106. Thus, in 1938, bacteria recovered from the hands were divided into two categories: transient and resident. Transient flora, which colonizes the superficial layers of the skin, is more amenable to removal by routine handwashing. HCWs often acquire them during direct contact with patients or contact with contaminating environmental surfaces in close proximity to a patient. Transient flora are organisms most frequently associated with infections. Resident flora, which are attached to deeper layers of the skin, are more resistant to removal. In addition, resident flora (e.g., coagulase-negative staphylococci and diphtheroids) are less likely to be associated with such infections. The hands of HCWs may become persistently colonized with pathogenic flora (e.g., *S. aureus*, gram-negative bacilli, or yeast). Investigators have documented that although the number of transient and resident flora varies considerably from person to person, it is often relatively consistent for any specific person (Boyce, Pittet 2002).

Cross Contamination in Private Homes

Mazengia, Fisk, Liao, Huang, and Meschike implemented a study in 2015 that used a combination approach, involving video-recorded observations of food-handling activities and questionnaires to assess food safety knowledge and declared practices. Thus, the investigation showed that 100% of participants reported washing their hands before preparation of meals, yet only 5% of the observed participants washed their hands. While 98% of participants reported that they washed their hands with soap and hot water after handling raw poultry, the observations found that hands were properly washed only 12% of the time, after being directly contaminated with raw chicken (Mazengia, Fisk, Liao, Huang, and Meschike 2015).

Thus, previous observational studies have reported a lack of proper handwashing practices among food handlers. An observational study evaluating the frequency of handwashing before, during, and after poultry meal preparation found that in only 5% of households were hands washed before beginning meal preparation, 35% after contact with raw poultry, and 5% after completing meal preparation. Thus, proper handwashing compliance is only approximately one-third the rate reported previously (Mazengia, Fisk, Liao, Huang, and Meschike 2015).

Further, apart from the lack of handwashing, the recommended duration of 20 seconds (s) of handwashing with soap and water is frequently not met. In this study, the length of handwashing with soap and hot water varied from as short as 2 s to as long as 33 s, with an overall average of 13 s (SD = 7; Mazengia, Fisk, Liao, Huang, and Meschike 2015). The CDC has set standards for handwashing. Hands should be washed and scrubbed for at least 20 s, as the "Happy Birthday" song is hummed twice. It is the best way to prevent illnesses and save lives (CDC 2016). Indeed, many researchers have investigated handwashing compliance and relationships to germs, sickness, and death over the years: Gibson and Markovic, D. (2015); Battistella G., et al., (2017); Jones R. et al., (2000); Gerberding, J. L. (2002); Mazengia, E., et al.,(2015); Bjerke, N. B. (2004); Burusnykyl, P. and Broz, C. C. (2013); Mathur, P. (2011); Pragle, A. S., Harding, K. A., and Mank, J. C. (2007); Teare, L. et al.,(2000); Pyrek, K. M. (2004); Mathur, P. (2011); Ellingson, K., at al., (2014); Garrett, J. H. (2013); Williams (2008); Stone, S. P. (2001); Sender, R., Fuchs, S. and Milo, R. (2016); and the United States Department of Labor, who assures the safety and healthful working conditions for working men and women.

However, the majority of the studies investigated have some limitations. One of the restrictions is that most of the studies are within healthcare facilities. Cross-contamination is prevalent in and should include other public industries, such as restaurants, since many individuals do not know the lack of handwashing and uncleanness passed on to them in various establishments. Thus, another limitation is the lack of surveillance. In order to ensure that people are washing their hands, direct observation is essential, because many individuals do not wash their hands or do not wash them appropriately, according to the CDC. Surveillance by camera has its limitations as well and can be misleading. Hence, Sahay et al. (2010) suggested that to obtain the most accurate data pertaining to handwashing compliance, direct observation should be viewed as the "gold standard." On the contrary, according to Gul et al. (2012), while direct observation is a more accurate measure, it requires more time, resources, and costs.

Summary

With the continuous growth of bacteria in this era, it is no surprise that drug resistance is at its critical peak. Hence, adding to this already crucial issue is the lack of handwashing that causes many individuals to become sick or even die. The healthcare field is not the only environment battling cross-contamination due to the lack of handwashing. Therefore, the controversy must be taken seriously and brought to the forefront, to ensure individuals are aware of possible reasons they or someone they know has become ill. The CDC declares that keeping one's hands clean through improved hand hygiene is one of the most important steps one can take to avoid getting sick or spreading germs to others, and that many diseases and conditions are spread by not washing one's hands with soap and clean running water. Thus, if clean running water is not accessible, as is common in many parts of the world, people should use soap and available water. If unavailable, people should use an alcohol-based hand sanitizer that contains at least 60% alcohol to clean their hands (CDC 2016). In order to decrease cross-contamination, it is highly necessary to examine and improve handwashing compliance rates as, contrary to common belief, handwashing compliance is surprisingly lower than expected (Gibson and Markovic 2015).

Table 1. Summary of observations for hand hygiene adherence measurement, including strengths and weaknesses.

Observation method	Strengths	Weaknesses
Direct observation	• Gold standard for hand hygiene adherence • Only method that can discern all opportunities for hand hygiene within patient care encounter and assess hand hygiene technique • Allows for immediate corrective feedback	• Labor intensive and costly Observers must be trained and validated • Subject to Hawthorne effect • Subject to selection and observer bias
Technology-assisted direct observation	• Use of technology (e.g., tablet computer) to save data entry step or to assist the observer in standardizing measurement (i.e., removing subjectivity) • Video-assisted observations can provide an assessment of all or most opportunities to be analyzed at a remote location • Less time-consuming and costly than direct observation	Requires investment and maintenance of infrastructure Video monitoring requires trained observers, has limited opportunity for immediate feedback, and has potential to impact patient privacy

Observation method	Strengths	Weaknesses
Product volume or event count measurement	• Not subject to Hawthorne effect or selection or observer bias • Unobtrusive and encompasses all opportunities • Counters can detect changes in frequency of use according to time of day or patterns of use in a hospital unit • May assist in optimal location of dispensers	• Relies on accurate usage data, which may be compromised by system gaps or intentional tampering • Cannot distinguish hand hygiene opportunities (no denominator) or who used the product • Cannot assess adequacy of technique • There are significant costs associated with event counting systems, and ongoing maintenance is required
Advanced technologies for automated monitoring	• Systems with wearable components can provide positive feedback or just-in-time reminders to perform hand hygiene and individual level monitoring • Captures all episodes entering and leaving a patient zone • (eliminating selection and observer bias) and associated adherence	• Expensive to implement and requires ongoing maintenance for all devices (e.g., battery replacement or recharging) • Difficult to detect opportunities within the patient encounter • or to assess technique • Concerns about healthcare worker privacy • Limited data outside of research settings

Observation method	Strengths	Weaknesses
Self-report	• Can raise individuals' awareness of their practice	• Unreliable as healthcare personnel overestimate their performance; should not be used for hand hygiene monitoring data (Ellingson et al. 2014).

Observation method	Strengths	Weaknesses
Self-report	• Can raise individuals'	• Unreliable as healthcare

CHAPTER 3

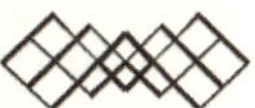

Methodology

Introduction

High-quality handwashing should be an acceptable norm for daily living to reduce the spread of infections that result in sickness and death. Thus, several authors of a study to prevent healthcare-associated infections through handwashing sponsored by Society for Healthcare Epidemiology of America(SHEA), Infectious Diseases Society of America (IDSA) and other experts in the field, convey the same message, as discussed in many other investigations and throughout this book, that hand hygiene is touted as one of the most important measures to prevent the transmission of infections in the community and healthcare settings. Close observations are the primary methods to investigate compliance with proper handwashing, and various other practices are utilized to study the relationship between hand hygiene and infections. Hence, for generations, handwashing with soap and water has been considered a measure of personal health (Boyce 2002). The concept of cleaning one's hands with antiseptics agents probably emerged in the early nineteenth century, as early as 1822; a French pharmacist demonstrated that solutions containing chlorides of lime or soda indicated that the foul odor associated solutions could be used as disinfectants and antiseptics (Boyce 2002).

In 1961, the US Public Health Service produced a training film that demonstrated handwashing techniques recommended for use by HCWs. Thus, at that time, personnel were directed to wash their hands with soap and water for 1–2 minutes, before and after patient contact. Rinsing hands with an antiseptic agent was believed to be less efficient than handwashing with soap and water. Additionally, antiseptic agents were recommended only in emergencies or in areas where sinks were unavailable (Boyce 2002).

Moreover, in 1975 and 1985, formally written CDC guidelines recommend handwashing with antimicrobial soap between contacts. Hence, these recommendations have been studied; therefore, cause for persons to have an understanding of healthy bacterial skin flora and models of hand transmission (CDC 2002).

Models of Hand Transmission

Several investigators have studied transmission of infectious agents using different experimental models. In one study, nurses were asked to touch the groins of patients heavily colonized with gram-negative bacilli for 15 seconds, with the gram as though they were taking a femoral pulse. Nurses then cleaned their hands by washing with plain soap and water or by using an alcohol hand rinse. After cleaning their hands, they touched a piece of urinary catheter material with their finger, and the catheter segment was cultured. The study revealed that touching intact areas of the patient's moist skin transferred enough organisms to the nurses' hands to result in subsequent transmission to the catheter material, despite handwashing with plain soap and water. It has also been found that organisms are transferred to various types of surfaces in much larger numbers (i.e., $> 10^4$) from wet hands than from hands that are thoroughly dried (Boyce and Pitt 2002).

Therefore, the pressing issue concerning infection control and the critical point to practice good hand hygiene is to investigate the standard practices for prevention and elimination of disease and death. On the contrary, for this book, several subsequent studies concerning the problem will be employed to understand:

I.   Handwashing behaviors
II. Professional habits of hand hygiene
III. Strategies to prevent infections through hand hygiene

Research Questions and Hypotheses

The studies for review should answer some important questions to help understand how to eliminate cross-contamination:

I.   Will hand hygiene prevent infections?
II. Are handwashing practices related to behaviors?
III. Is hand rubbing with an alcohol-based solution more efficient in reducing hand contamination than handwashing with soap and water?

> H1a: Those who utilize good hand hygiene contribute to the prevention of infections.
> H1o: Those who utilize good hand hygiene are less likely to prevent infections.
> H2a: The practice of handwashing could be related to behaviors.
> H2o: The practice of handwashing is not related to behavior.
> H3a: Hand rubbing with alcohol-based solutions may be more effective in reducing hand contamination than washing with soap and water.

This study will utilize three studies that examine the critical need for handwashing.

Study One: Strategies to Prevent Healthcare-Associated Infections through Hand Hygiene (2014)

Researchers Girou, Loyeau, Legrand, Oppein, and BrunBuisson conducted a prospective randomized clinical trial with blinded evaluation of microbiological results. It was performed from June to July 2000 in three intensive care units (two surgical and one medical) of a 940-bed tertiary care facility and a referral university hospital. Eligible HCWs were permanent and temporary nurses and nursing assistants of each unit. If any of the workers refused to participate, an alternative person was enrolled (Girou et al., 2002).

Treatment Groups

At the beginning of each session, when each participant arrived at the unit (7:00 a.m.), opaque sealed envelopes were used to assign him or her randomly to standard handwashing with a medicated soap (chlorhexidine gluconate, 4%; Hibiscrub; Zeneca Pharma) or hand-rubbing with a waterless alcohol-based solution (45% 2-propanol; 30% 1-propanol; 0.2% mecetronium ethyl sulfate, average 3–5 mL; Sterillium; Bode Chemie; Hamburg; Germany). All participants had been previously instructed in the use of the alcohol-based solution when the hospital-wide hand-rubbing policy was launched a year prior by the infection control committee (Girou, Loyeau, Legrand, Oppein, and Buisson 2002).

A written protocol was available in each unit, and no additional information was provided to the participants before the study began. The sole exclusion criterion was applied to those participants who were assigned to handwashing but whose hands became visibly soiled (such as with body fluids). They then had to wash their hands with a standard antiseptic soap, and the session was ceased (Girou, Loyeau, Legrand, Oppein, and Buisson 2002)

Monitoring and Data Collection

Patient care activities were monitored during daily sessions of two to three hours until a predetermined number of eligible activities had been performed (see figure 1). One session comprised five patients' care activities that required hand hygiene before and after, which corresponded to 10 hand samples (five samples obtained beforehand cleaning and five after). Eligible activities were being in direct contact with the skin of a patient before invasive care, after interruption of care, and after contact with any part of a patient that was colonized with multi-resistant bacteria. The recording of the types of care performed, duration of care, whether participants wore gloves, number of opportunities for hand hygiene according to the recent guidelines, number of actual hand hygiene procedures performed, and duration of hand hygiene procedure (i.e., duration of use of the antiseptic agent; Girou, Loyeau, Legrand, Oppein, and Buisson 2002) were maintained.

Study Two: Strategies to Prevent Healthcare-Associated Infections through Hand Hygiene (2014); Methods for Hand Hygiene Adherence Measurement

Ellingson, Haas, Aiello, Kusek et al. (2014) highlighted practical recommendations with the current scientific evidence for hand hygiene. Hence, the primary hand hygiene measurement methods were direct observation, indirect volume or event count measurement, and advanced technologies for automated adherence monitoring. Each method had strengths and weaknesses. Using multiple methods to measure hand hygiene is a way to address the strengths and limitations associated with a single-measurement approach. Gould et al. recommended that the feasibility and acceptability of a combined approach should be explored with further studies to refine the method.

Direct Observation

Direct observation included in-person monitoring of hand hygiene behavior. Thus, to enhance the validity and reliability of direct observation, it is crucial that observers are properly trained, and that their views are validated initially and at intervals to ensure accuracy. The WHO have developed a suite of tools to help standardize the observation process. To minimize the Hawthorne effect, or behavior change based on participants' awareness of being observed, some facilities have used covert observers or "secret shoppers." Although the use of hidden observers may improve the validity of the measurement and be appropriate for quality improvement initiatives, some experts have raised ethical concerns about avoiding informed consent of those being observed. Furthermore, it is unlikely that the covert nature of the observations can be sustained (Ellingson et al. 2014).

Some protocols used by direct observers provide immediate feedback for noncompliant observations (i.e., "just-in-time training") or document the names of noncompliant individuals, making the observation part of the intervention. This is appropriate for the goal of increasing hand hygiene, but adherence is likely to be inflated by the presence of an observer who is collecting names or providing feedback. Observer and selection bias are the systematic inclusion of selected opportunities, nurses focus on the behavior of physicians and vice versa or only observing certain shifts), which may be minimized by randomizing audit times and directing observers to observe a minimum number of opportunities across healthcare personnel (HCP) types (Ellingson et al. 2014).

There was no accepted standard stipulating the number and distribution of hand hygiene opportunities that facilities or units should observe. Poor hand hygiene is likely to be revealed with fewer observations. Seeing good adherence in a tiny sample of opportunities, however, is less reassuring. Reports of hand hygiene adherence are often called into question because of the perceived inadequacy in number or representativeness of observations to reflect true adherence. A study documenting every entry and exit opportunity over a 14-day period found that a simulated observer placed in the ward for 1 hour could have observed a minimal number of opportunities; however, if simulated observers switched locations every 15 minutes, more opportunities and a greater diversity of HCP could be observed. Another study showed that observers placed at a greater physical distance from the observed hand hygiene opportunities made more errors, as did observers on wards with higher activity levels (Ellingson, Haas, Aiello, Kusek, Maragakis, Olmsted, and Yoko 2014)

Indirect Hand Hygiene Adherence through Volume or Event Count Measurement

Product usage (soap, alcohol-based hand rub [ABHR]) or dispenser use is an indirect measurement of hand hygiene adherence and can be used to monitor trends in consumption over time or by type of care unit. This can be as simple as tracking the amount of product used by individual groups over time. Product usage can also be compared with the industry-average volume of a single dose of product when estimating adherence rates. Product measurement can be hampered by unreliable usage data from distribution, materials management, intentional tampering with dispensers, or a deliberate waste of product (Ellingson, Haas, Aiello, Kusek, Maragakis, Olmsted, and Yokoe 2014).

There are also advanced dispenser-based counters that create a date and time stamp each time the dispenser is used. Counting devices can also be placed into personal dispensers of ABHR worn on the body to increase the convenience of hand hygiene. In some studies, increased use of ABHR was associated with an increase in observed hand hygiene adherence; however, not all studies have found such an association. Automated dispenser counting systems may cost upwards of $30,000–40,000 per patient care unit, and data must be manually downloaded from the counters if an automatic web-based download via Wi-Fi is not used. Additionally, the counters must be monitored for low battery signals and disappearance by unauthorized persons (Ellingson et al., 2014).

Study Three: Drivers and Motivators in Consumer Handwashing Behavior (2014)

Burusnukul and Broz conducted a study at a university in the American Southwest in the health service department to determine the handwashing behaviors of students, faculty, and staff. In 2012, researchers conducted a traditional online survey embedded in a university-wide weekly electronic newsletter. Both students and employees at the participating university were recruited for the study. The sample represented members of the community with potential exposure to the handwashing promotion campaign (Clean Hand Campaign) as well as the health risks associated with different sanitation practices among members of a public institution (Burusnukul and Broz 2013).

The Clean Hands Campaign is a significant study because it has aided in the promotion materials (5"×5" posters) in all public restrooms on the university campus since 2008. The posters were placed above the handwashing sinks, inside the restroom door visible to the users as they exit, and on the interior walls of the restrooms. The poster provided a simple reminder for the university community to wash their hands: "Have you washed your hands 2day?" In a separate attempt to promote public health, the university also provided wall-mounted alcohol-based hand-sanitizer dispensers in limited buildings (Burusnukul and Broz 2013).

Data were collected between February and May of 2012 using an online self-report survey via SurveyMonkey.com. Both students and employees at the participating university were recruited for the study. The sample represented members of the community with potential exposure to the handwashing promotion campaign as described above, as well as to the health risks associated with varying sanitation practices among members of a public institution (Burusnukul and Broz 2013).

To assess university students' and employees' beliefs about handwashing, there were five beliefs associated with handwashing applicable to the study context, as follows:

I. Protecting oneself and others from getting sick
II. Influencing the handwashing behavior of others
III. Feeling good about oneself as doing the right thing.
IV. Hands becoming dry, cracked, and reddened.
V. Wasting a lot of time

Construction of belief items followed Ajzen's (2006) instructions and regarded each behavioral belief as comprising two parts: the behavioral belief strength and outcome evaluation. Together, the five behavioral belief item pairs were used to produce aggregate scores in assessing university students' and employees' attitudes toward handwashing behaviors.

Both subjective and objective knowledge regarding handwashing performance were measured. Subjective experience was measured using seven statements rated on a five-point Likert scale, with 1 representing "strongly disagree" and 5 representing "strongly agree." Of the seven items, four were adapted from the Subjective Knowledge Scale used in consumer behavior research (Flynn and Goldsmith 1999) and three were added to address the "why, when, and how" of proper handwashing. To measure objective knowledge, participants were asked to respond to four test questions relating to hand sanitization and handwashing procedures.

Summary

Past and present researchers have emphasized the critical need to inhibit the growth and spread of infection-causing bacteria. Hence, handwashing is one of the primary ways in which individuals can prevent transmission of bacteria that results in disease or even death.

There is an increase in bacteria that cause adverse, unfavorable reactions in the human body that have become resistant to some antibiotics. This means that, some individuals are not aware of or are not concerned about the nonimmunity to diseases, analytical research, or the predicament that bacteria may factor in humankind.

The issue has come to the point where researchers are advising people to avoid handshakes. In an article written by the Statesmen Newspaper (2002), it is indicated that one does not need to be coughed or sneezed upon by a cold sufferer to pick up a virus; sometimes, the process is more insidious. For example, someone touches his or her runny nose, then shake your hand, and you touch your nose or rub your eyes. Thus, you have caught a cold. Of course, touching or scratching your nose will not directly put a cold virus into the nasopharynx, but a virus deposited at the base of the nose can easily be inhaled into the nose. Additionally, the virus can gain entry via the tear ducts. Therefore, it is essential for people to wash their hands often and utilize soap and water (*Statesman*, New Delhi 2002).

Lulled by the success of antibiotics, Americans have come to think of compulsory handwashing as a thing of the past—a holdover from the sterile, hyper-hygienic 1950s. However, more than half the staph infections caught by hospital patients are now resistant to methiocillin (up from 2% in 1974), and according to some epidemiologists, the deaths of four children in Minnesota and North Dakota, infected by Staphylococcus Aureus, a bacterium that is easily passed through hand contact should bring an alert (Williams III, 2005).

Hence, Ralph Cordell, an epidemiologist at the CDC in Atlanta, stated, "handwashing is the most effective disease-preventing measure anyone can practice" (As cited in Williams, 1999). By all means, if one washes his or her hands, 95% of the organisms would be wiped out (Williams 1999).

Furthermore, the studies utilized in this investigation have provided great insight into how to set up infection programs to prevent infections, handwashing observations, and inhibit cross-contamination. Thus, continuous research can and will lead to educating others concerning this vital issue. Giroy, Loyeu, Legrand, Oppein, and Brun-Buisson shared some essential data when they compared the efficacy of hand-rubbing with an alcohol-based solution versus conventional handwashing with antiseptic soap and water to reduce hand contamination. Thus, since handwashing is the single most crucial step to prevent cross contamination, an alcohol-based solution would be the next best, when a sink, soap, and water are unavailable (Giroy, Loyeu, Legrand, Oppein, and Brun-Buisson 2002).

Thus, other authors, such as Ellingson, et al., (2014) have studied strategies to prevent defilement and assist healthcare facilities in implementing hand hygiene programs that are professional, scientific, and evidence-based. Indeed, knowledge will enhance handwashing skills and bring about an understanding of cross-contamination.

Finally, Burusnukul and Broz's investigation leads in a somewhat different direction. Researchers investigated drivers and motivations in consumer handwashing behaviors. They posted signs in various places throughout a university campus and observed students, faculty, and staff washing their hands after using the lavatories (Burusnukul and Broz 2013).

CHAPTER 4

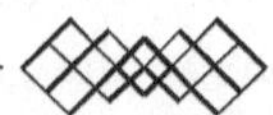

Results

Introduction

Handwashing is a critical topic to explore. Information presented in previous research to assist in the reduction and/or elimination of infections was identified in this review study. Hence, the information obtained during the investigation contains some vital results to educate the public and wage war—and win—against a variety of infectious organisms that cause sickness and even death (Turkoski 2005). Three studies were investigated to obtain the best information that will effectively educate and encourage others in relation to infection control and the critical need to wash one's hands. The results of the studies indicate the lack of handwashing among various groups, the essential need to implement evidence-based hand hygiene programs, and common handwashing behaviors. The results should answer the questions and hypotheses above related to cross-contamination and hand hygiene.

Findings from Study One

Handwashing is the primary action that must be taken to kill germs. In the first study, researchers compared the efficacy of hand rubbing with an alcohol-based solution versus conventional handwashing with antiseptic soap in reducing hand contamination. A total of 23 HCWs were included; 12 were randomized to hand rubbing and 11 were handwashing (fig. 1). Randomized participants performed 114 patient care activities (59 in the hand-rubbing group and 55 in the handwashing group). The distribution of events was comparable between the two groups. Table 1 shows the baseline characteristics of the two randomized groups and the activities performed. Gloves were worn during most events with a similar frequency between groups (Girou, Loyeau, Legrand, Oppein, and Brun-Buisson 2002).

In both groups, bacterial counts were lower after hand hygiene (Table 2). Figure 2 shows that for each participant the median reduction of bacterial contamination achieved by hand rubbing was significantly higher than the reduction achieved by handwashing (83% [interquartile range 78% –92%] vs. 58% [58% –74%], respectively, $P=0.012$). Hence, the difference in the percentage reduction between the two groups was 26% (95% confidence interval 8% to 44%) (Girou, Loyeau, Legrand, Oppein, and Brun-Buisson 2000). During the monitoring sessions, the median cumulative number of observed hand-rubbed was 1 (0–3) before the first sample and 10 (6–14) before the fifth sample. The percentage reduction in contamination at the first evaluated hand rubbing was 88% (74% –97%), and at the fifth was 95% (76% –99%). By all means, hand-rubbing remained effective after several applications of the alcohol-based solution. The median time spent on hand hygiene was relatively low in the handwashing group, where the antiseptic soap was applied for only 30 seconds (23–37 seconds); 36 handwashing procedures (65%) lasted less than 30 seconds. Thus, the median duration of hand-rubbing was also 30 seconds (29–33 seconds), which is the required time for bactericidal activity. (Girou, Loyeau, Legrand, Oppein, and BrunBuisson 2000).

Microbiological Samples and Processing

When there was an opportunity for hand hygiene, an imprint of fingertips and palm occurred from the participant's dominant hand before and one minute after the procedure. Thus, if the participant wore gloves during the procedure, the gloves were removed before the sample was collected. Each fingertip and palm were pressed onto commercial contact agar plates (one plate per finger and one per palm) that contained neutralizers (lecithin, polysorbate 80, sodium thiosulfate, Count-Tact, BioMerieux, SA, Marcy I'Etoile, France). Plates were incubated at 37°C under aerobic conditions. Additionally, the total bacterial contamination of the hands was recorded as the number of colony forming units (cfu) recovered from both the fingertips and palm after 48 hours of intubation. The precise count up was evaluated to a maximum of 300 cfu, as colonies formed a confluent growth. The bacteria identified were Staphylococcus aureus or other pathogenic bacteria not usually found in skin flora, by using standard microbiological procedures and their susceptibility to antibiotics was determined. MRSA as mentioned is the most prevalent multi-resistant organism. There were no anaerobic cultures. A preliminary test was performed to assess the practical neutralization of each tested product using a suspension of 10^4 MRSA per ml. Two observers (SL and FO) were responsible for the entire protocol (monitoring and sampling) in all units. They stayed in the unit without interfering with hand hygiene (that is, the quality of hand hygiene), whatever method was used (Girou, Loyeau, Legrand, Oppein, and Buisson 2002).

Statistical Analysis

The analysis was based on the intention to treat disease; one participant dropped out of the study after four samplings instead of five because his hands were visibly soiled with body fluids. The participants were the units of analysis. The bacterial counts were expressed as numbers of cfu per hand. First, the percentage reduction was calculated in hand contamination for each cleaning procedure. Second, the average percentage reduction was obtained for each participant by calculating the mean of the five methods per participant and using Mann–Whitney U tests to compare the percentage reduction between the groups. The summary statistics on the bacterial counts were means and standard deviations (SD) with 95% confidence intervals, medians, and interquartile ranges. To perform the analysis and consider $P < 0.05$ as significant, epi-info 6.0 (CDC, Atlanta) was used (Girou, Loyeau, Legrand, Oppein, and Buisson 2002).*Figures 1-2:study to compare alcohol solution to handwashing by Girou, et, et al., 2002.

Figure *4.1

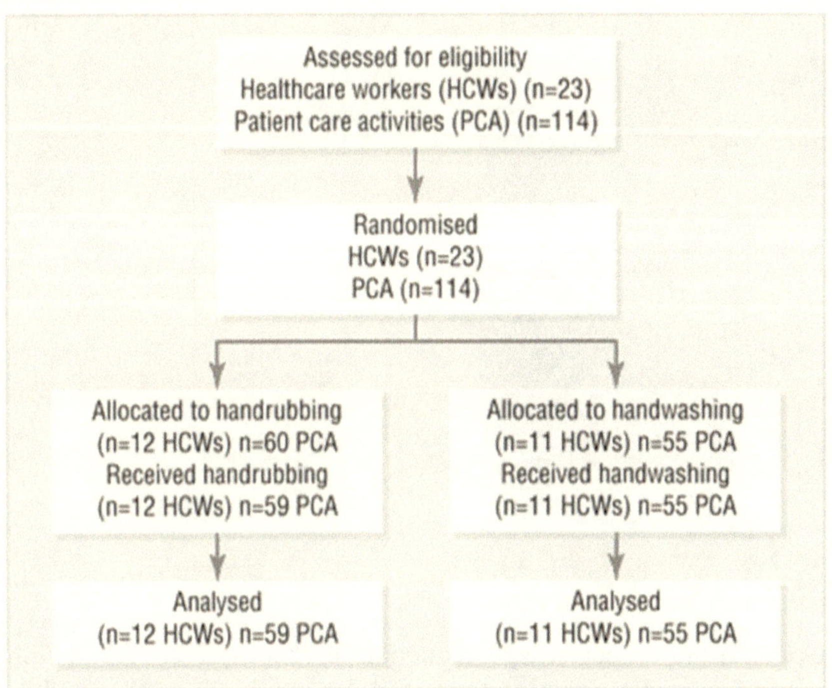

*Studies to compare alcohol solution to handwashing by Girou, et, et al., 2002.

Schematic schedule of monitoring sampling sessions (one participant allocated to hand-rubbing did not use it on one occasion, because of visible soiling with body fluids—the sole contraindication for using alcohol-based solutions.)

Figure *4.2

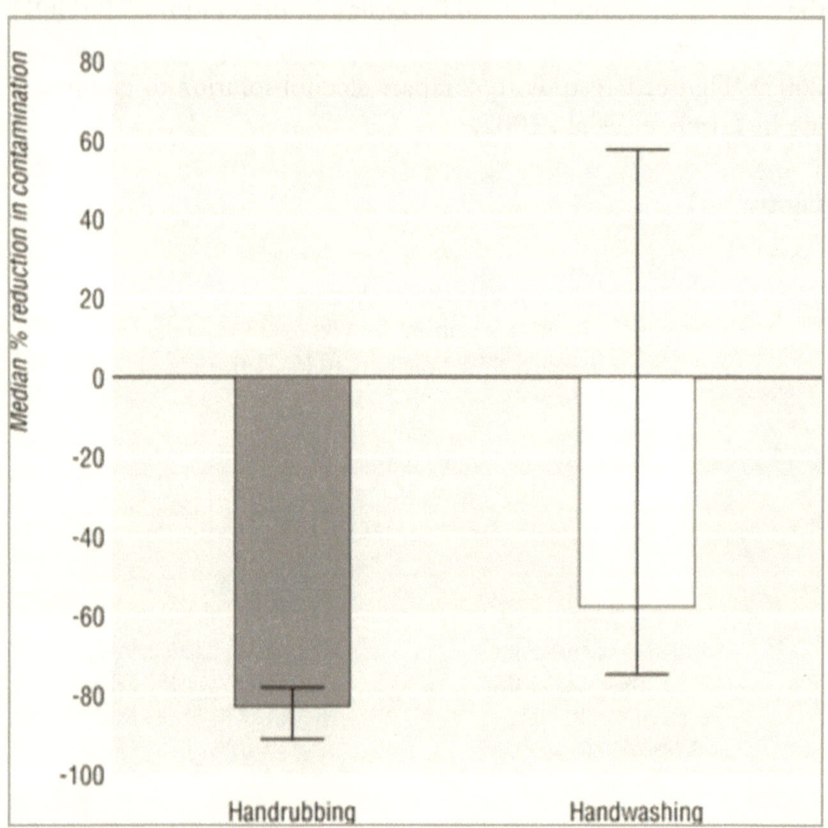

Comparison of percentage reduction in bacterial contamination of participants' hands obtained after hand-rubbing with an alcohol-based solution or after handwashing with antiseptic soap. Results were expressed as a median and interquartile range; the difference between the two groups was significant (P = 0.012).

Table *4.1 Characteristics of two groups of HCWs randomized to hand-rubbing with alcohol-based solution or handwashing

	Hand-rubbing (n=12)	Handwashing (n=11)
Nurses	5	6
Nursing assistants	6	3
Nursing students	1	2
No of patient care activities included	59	55
Median (IQR) duration of patient care activities (min)	11 (5–20)	15 (7–25)
No (%) activities when gloves were worn	51 (86)	46 (83)
Cumulative No (IQR) of hand hygiene procedures performed during monitoring sessions	11 (7–15)	8 (7–13)
Median (IQR) duration of monitoring sessions (min)	91 (58–177)	75 (35–132)
No of opportunities observed	184	158
Proportion (95% CI) compliance with hand hygiene	71 (45–96)	64 (36–93)

- IQR=interquartile range Table 4.1 By Girou, et al.,(2002)

*Table 4.2 Bacterial counts (colony forming units) before and after two methods of hand cleaning.

	Before		After		Median % reduction (IQR)
	Mean (SD); 95% CI	Median (IQR)	Mean (SD); 95% CI	Median (IQR)	
Hand-rubbing	271 (372); 174 to 368	101 (29–380)	35 (59); 20 to 50	7 (2–31)	86 (70–96)
Handwashing	232 (331); 143 to 321	117 (15–239)	69 (106); 41 to 97	9 (1–135)	73 (25–93)

- IQR = interquartile range. * By Girou, et al.,(2002)

Study Two: Strategies to Prevent Healthcare-associated Infections through Hand Hygiene

This investigation was an in-depth examination to help healthcare organizations implement hand hygiene programs and highlight some recommendations for the program. The author of the text discusses strategies to prevent cross-contamination. Hence, they utilize a professional scientific evidence-based approach to assist healthcare personnel in preventing the spread of infections (Elling, Haas, Aiello, Kusek, Maragakis, Olmsted, and Yokoe 2014). Indeed, there is an abundance of tools and methods for monitoring and reporting hand hygiene adherence from direct observation, to volume-based measurements, to emerging automated oversight technologies. However, it is essential to share the results of the hand hygiene strategies that were directly and indirectly observed.

Direct Observation

The observations of this study entail overseeing every entry and exit opportunity over a 14-day period, and a simulated observer was placed on a ward for 1 hour could have observed a very small number of opportunities. However, if simulated observers switched locations every 15 minutes, more opportunities and a greater diversity of HCP types could be seen. In a similar study, observers who were placed at a more significant physical distance from the observed hand hygiene opportunities made more errors, as did observers on wards with higher activity levels (Elling, Haas, Aiello, Kusek, Maragakis, Olmsted, and Yokoe 2014).

Indirect Observation

These observations resulted in many hindrances. Hence, it was found that results can be hampered by unreliable usage data from intentional tampering with dispensers or deliberately wasting products. Additionally, the counter must be monitored for low battery signals and disappearance; with the addition of the cost of an automated system, it can be expensive to operate. The price could range from $30,000–40,000 per-patient care unit (Elling, Haas, Aiello, Kusek, Maragakis, Olmsted, and Yokoe 2014).

Overview

Due to the reasons discussed above, although this study investigated direct and indirect methods of observing handwashing, as mentioned earlier, the study had other ways to monitor and report hand hygiene. Hence, some of the reviews were conducted to investigate hand hygiene product efficacy, such as efficacy versus bacteria, effectiveness versus viruses, efficiency based on dispensing mechanism, technique, and tolerability.

1. Efficacy versus Bacteria

In the studies conducted to compare the relative efficacy of various hand hygiene products against bacteria, the majority of the reviews, ABHRs (with alcohol concentrations between 62% and 95%) are described as being more effective than either plain or antimicrobial soaps over a broad range of testing conditions. There were 13 clinical studies of hand hygiene product efficacy against bacteria that compared ABHR with soap products in use by HCP. Of these, 12 reported ABHR to be superior to soap formulations, and 1 reported equivalence of ABHR with soap products (Elling, Haas, Aiello, Kusek, Maragakis, Olmsted, and Yokoe 2014).

2. Efficacy versus Viruses

Many of the available studies show that ABHRs have significantly better efficacy in removing several different viruses than both non-antimicrobial and antimicrobial soap and water, suggesting that ABHRs are likely to provide some protection against several respiratory and enteric viruses on the hands. Hence, more studies are necessary to identify the best formulations for inactivation of microorganisms on the hands of HCP (Elling, Haas, Aiello, Kusek, Maragakis, Olmsted, and Yokoe 2014).

3.   Efficacy Based on Dispensing Mechanism

The 2002 CDC guidelines state that "alcohol-containing hand wipes were not a substitute for gel or foam ABHRs, on the basis of "inferior efficacy"(p. 943). Since then, alcohol-containing wipes have been reported to have similar efficacy to ABHR gel and foam against influenza virus. It appears that some formulations of alcohol-based wipes with at least 65% alcohol are now comparable to alcohols delivered by other dispensing methods. Moreover, it was found that alcohol-containing hand wipes offer a convenient option for bed-bound patients, first responders, and others who cannot quickly reach a sink or wall dispenser (Elling, Haas, Aiello, Kusek, Maragakis, Olmsted, and Yokoe 2014).

4.   Technique

The minimum time recommended and required by the CDC for handwashing is 15–20 seconds. The hand hygiene volume necessary changes based on the size of one's hands to meet the time requirement. However, recent studies suggest that 15 seconds is insufficient for meeting standards for high-quality hand disinfection (EN 1500)[122] (Elling, Haas, Aiello, Kusek, Maragakis, Olmsted, and Yokoe 2014).

Study Three: Drivers and Motivators in Consumer Handwashing Behavior

This handwashing study was regulated by a university to investigate behaviors toward the effectiveness of handwashing. Hence, signs were placed ubiquitously on campus to remind students, faculty, and staff to wash their hands. A total of 186 respondents (62.8% female and 37.2% male) completed the survey. Participants included students (49.2%), faculty (15.8%), administrators (3.3%), support staff (23.5%), and others (8.2%). Ages ranged from 19 to 80 years (M = 37.49). All ethnic groups were represented in the sample, with the majority being white/non-Hispanic (67.8%) and Hispanic (21.7%; Burusnukul and Broz 2013).

The results indicated that participants generally believed in the positive outcomes of handwashing practices, including the following:

I.   Protecting oneself and others from getting sick (M = 4.41)
II. Influencing others to do the same (M = 3.54)
III. Feeling good about oneself as doing the right thing (M = 3.96)

Furthermore, they did not agree that handwashing practices would result in adverse outcomes, including the following:

I.   Wasting a lot of time (M = 1.74)
II. Hands became dry, cracked, and reddened (M = 2.57); however, they believed that these outcomes were decidedly undesirable, as reported in the outcome evaluations (M = 1.84 and M = 2.05, respectively; Burusnukul and Broz 2013).

In assessing the overall results of attitudes toward handwashing behavior, the aggregate score was derived from the sum of multiplicative products of the five behavioral belief item pairs. Of the five behavioral belief strength statements, two connoted adverse outcomes of handwashing: "If I wash my hands whenever I should, I will be dry, cracked, and reddened." Therefore, reverse scoring was applied to these statements (Burusnukul and Broz 2013).

The values of aggregate attitude scores of could range from 5 to 125, with 45 being the determinant score (i.e., neutral in all counts), differentiating between positive and negative opinions. The results showed aggregate scores for mentality ranging from 17 to 110, with a mean of 67.70. The majority of participants (93.5%) reported positive attitudes toward handwashing practices (i.e., scores above 45) (Burusnukul and Broz 2013).

As for self-reported hand sanitization practices, participants relied more on handwashing than using alcohol-based sanitizer to sanitize their hands in all instances. Table 1 shows the averages of both the number of handwashes performed and alcohol-based hand sanitizer used for each of the scenarios (Burusnukul and Broz 2013).

When evaluating the relationship of predisposing factors (beliefs, attitude, and knowledge) and self-reported handwashing performance, the aggregate (summed) handwashing performance score was computed for the ten scenarios where handwashing was necessary. The results of Pearson r correlation analysis are presented in Table 2 (Burusnukul and Broz 2013)

Of the five beliefs about handwashing, only the idea that handwashing would lead to hands becoming dry, cracked, and reddened was not significantly related to handwashing performance. Results suggested a positive relationship between attitude and handwashing performance (r = 0.312, p < 0.01). A similar association was found between subjective knowledge and handwashing performance (r = 4.415, p < 0.01), but not for objective knowledge *(Burusnukul and Broz 2013).

*Table 4. 3. Self-reported hand sanitization practices by Burusnukul & Broz 2013

Hand sanitization scenarios	Handwashing		Alcohol-based	
	Performed		Sanitizer used	
	Mean	SD	Mean	SD
Before, during, and after preparing food	7.77	2.698	2.75	3.678
Before eating food	6.73	3.192	3.20	3.543
After touching garbage	8.05	3.104	3.10	3.851
After contact with an ill person or soiled materials such as tissues	8.09	2.992	3.74	3.881

Before and after treating a cut or wound	8.11	3.006	3.37	4.006
After changing diapers or cleaning up a child who has used the toilet	8.53	2.897	3.35	4.066
After touching an animal or animal waste	8.00	3.097	3.19	3.901
After you have touched your mouth, eyes, or any body parts	5.34	3.418	2.85	3.545
After blowing your nose, coughing, or sneezing	6.34	3.329	3.31	3.657
After you use the toilet	8.41	2.953	3.20	4.04

*Table 4.2. Correlations—predisposing factors and self-reported handwashing performance.

Predisposing factors Self-reported Handwashing Performance	Performance
If I wash my hands whenever I should, I will protect myself and others from getting sick	0.342*
If I wash my hands whenever I should, I will waste a lot of my time	0.343*
If I wash my hands whenever I should, they will be dry, cracked, and reddened	0.063*
If I wash my hands whenever I should, I will influence others to do the same	0.242*
If I wash my hands whenever I should, I will feel good about myself as doing the right thing	0.358*
Attitude	0.312*
Subjective knowledge	0.415*
Objective knowledge	0.118*
Note: *Correlation is significant at: *0.01 level*	
Correlations – predisposing factors and self-reported handwashing performance	

Summary

The effect brought about by washing or not washing one's hands has been observed in this chapter, from either the results of soap and water or hand-rubbing alcohol-based solutions. Hence, documentation is essential to view the outcomes of people who utilize good hand hygiene and those who do not.

Hence, many behaviors can determine the motivation to wash his or her hands. Indeed, whatever an individual's motives are for not appropriately washing his or her hands, this study should prevent with the certainty that notion that proper handwashing saves lives. Thus, educating and informing others about the dangers of not washing their hands can lead to a drastic change, thereby reducing disease transmission

The reviewed studies show that handwashing is key to the reduction of cross-contamination. The observation of lower bacterial counts after hand hygiene shows that clean hands reduce infections, resulting in fewer persons dying from disease. By all means, the war on infection must be stressed, as if one were about to ingest poison. Indeed, it seems common sense that hands should be washed, at least when visibly soiled. However, it is important to consider that invisible pathogens can reside on the hand's surface (Paez et al. 2007). Thus, washing hands properly and adequately helps to break the chain of circumstances that lead to potential disease transmission.

Notably, in relation to food preparation and consumption, contaminated hands can repeatedly transfer foodborne pathogens and increase the chances of cross-contamination from various contact surfaces to ready-to-eat foods (Kassa et al. 2001; Redmond et al. 2004). The CDC recommends that hands be washed before, during, and after food preparation, as well as before eating food (CDC 2012a; Burusnukul and Broz 2013).

In other instances where hands can become contaminated, handwashing is necessary before and after caring for someone who is sick, before and after treating a cut or wound, after using the toilet, after changing diapers or cleaning up a child who has used the bathroom, after blowing one's nose, coughing, or sneezing, after touching an animal or animal waste, after handling pet food or pet treats, and after touching garbage (CDC 2012a).

Descriptive statistics were employed to assess beliefs, attitudes, knowledge, and self-reported handwashing behavior as well as the awareness of the Clean Hands Campaign. Pearson's correlation and t-test analyses were conducted to evaluate the relationships between predisposing factors and self-reported handwashing behavior. To determine the effectiveness of the program, t-test analysis was performed to reveal any differences in handwashing practices between those who had and had not seen the Clean Hands Campaign post (Burusnykyl and Broz 2013).

Finally, the utilization of hand sanitizers as a convenient product can reduce microbial pathogens from the hand's surface; however, this is not an unconditional replacement for proper handwashing. Some viruses can resist physiochemical inactivation and require vigorous friction during handwashing to be removed from the hands (Michaels et al. 2004). Furthermore, the viscous nature of the gel may only provide a shield for the virus. This shield eventually wears off after repeated touching or handling, and transmission of pathogens can still occur with other surfaces and foods (Bidawid et al.200; Burusnukul and Broz 2013).

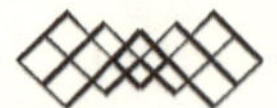

CHAPTER 5

Discussion, Conclusion, and Recommendations

Introduction

Infection control is an important issue in healthcare, but we must not forget that germs can be spread anywhere, if individuals do not practice good hand hygiene. Hence, the ones that know and understand the consequences of not practicing hand hygiene must take a stand, educate, and inform others of the critical need to wash their hands. This is a primary step to defeat cross-contamination and leave germs behind and/or destroyed.

Undeniably, we have the purpose of waging war and winning the battle against the lack of handwashing that leads to the transmission of a variety of infective organisms that bring harm. One must be aware that the chances of encountering contaminated objects and surfaces are heightened, especially in public places, since many objects in public areas are accessible to several users or are handled by unknown hands. However, one must remember that bacteria are everywhere, in the home and in restaurants. Therefore, it is essential to have a unified sense of responsibility to keep from contacting and spreading illness-causing pathogens. It is a primary concern to reduce the transmission of disease by washing one's hands. To reflect on the prior research questions and hypothesis, good hand hygiene is the ethical attitude toward infection control to prevent the spread of infections.

Conclusion

Evidence has shown that proper handwashing leads to a reduction in infections and saves lives. It is like watching out not only for one's self but also speaking up to remind others to wash their hands. Hands are indeed dirty, especially since throughout the day, they come into contact with various objects such as money, door knobs, and pets. Thus, one of my main concerns is that individuals must serve others. Hence, these examples are personal experiences. If one is handling money in a restaurant, by all means, do not prepare the food. Money is dirty and must be treated as such. In addition, when one visits the restroom, think about what is happening without stopping at the sink to utilize soap and water. There is significant transmission of bacteria from handling bathroom doors, using the commode, wiping self, and then returning to previous activities, without proper handwashing.

Furthermore, investigations on cross-contamination and hand hygiene have been researched, exposed, and broadcast ages back; however, it may not be enough since nosocomial infections and other illnesses that have been proved to be a result of the lack of handwashing are still at a peak. Reflecting on some of the secondary data utilized to investigate this report on controlling the spread of diseases by utilizing proper handwashing techniques. Thus, it has been centuries since humans learned the significance of hand hygiene. Some scholars have provided evidence that decontamination can markedly reduce the incidence of mortality. Thus, in the accumulation of data, as mentioned earlier in this book, the physician Semmelweis acquired a breakthrough concerning cross-contamination that resulted in policies for washing hands that also led to a tenfold decrease in the mortality rate (Mathur 2011).

Furthermore, for this writing, some information was beneficial in that the secondary data showed that direct contact was the primary mode of transmission of Staphylococcal Aureus epidemics. Indeed, the list of investigations and evidence obtained from materials gathered to write this book has given a considerable amount of ammunition or information to share and win the battle against cross-contamination. For instance, the evidence mentioned above and throughout this book were relevant material to share, especially for individuals that utilize hand sanitizers and those that do not. It was refreshing to learn that in customary conditions, hand-rubbing was at least as effective as handwashing with an antiseptic soap. Of course, there may be different opinions about hand-rubbing alcohol, soap, and water. Some testimonies say that hand-rubbing only shields the germs, and that the shield will soon evaporate. It is a debate that requires education in the healthcare arena as well as the public, but mainly the public, since HCWs are taught to wash hands with soap and water after utilizing the sanitizer a few times. By all means, some said there was nothing like soap and water. Otherwise, the sanitizer was the next best option. However, there were widely held beliefs concerning the consequences of handwashing behaviors (Clayton, Green, Selman, and Pragle 2007). Some participants had positive results, and some had negative beliefs about hand hygiene. This writing was concentrated on the positive concerns of proper hand hygiene, but later the negatives will be shared in the summary. Indeed, the positive beliefs about performing adequate handwashing include preventing communicable diseases and influencing others to engage in the same desired behavior (i.e., doing the right thing) must stay steady to save lives (Burusnukul and Broz 2013).

Of course, it is not always the best method to be openly honest and suspicious of those that may or may not have washed their hands. However, viewing the three studies utilized for this paper and researching other materials on the numbers and observations of individuals that do and those that do not comply with signs, rules, and regulations for infection control, there should not be any question about uniting to be watchful and utilizing standard precautions. However, the issues have gone beyond the usual care since some infections are resistant to several types of antibiotics, and some researchers have even suggested eliminating handshakes.

Inevitably, most believe that handwashing is essential to save lives. Therefore, handwashing should become an education priority, especially since numerous investigations have shown that handwashing reduces cross-contamination. Indeed, hand hygiene is the practice of evidence-based medicine. Therefore, programs to improve these methods are a way to educate decontaminating hands and substantially mitigate infections (Stone 2001).

Recommendations

Promotion of hand hygiene is a major challenge for infection control experts. In service education, the distribution of information leaflets, workshops and lectures, and performance feedback on compliance rates have been associated with transient improvement. However because of the complexity of the process of change, a multimodal, multidisciplinary strategy is necessary, especially since advanced technology is also means of improving cross-contamination (CDC 2001).

Improvement in infection control practices requires questioning basic beliefs, continuous assessment of the stages of behavioral change, interventions with an appropriate process of change, and supporting individual and group creativity (CDC 2001). To improve compliance with hand hygiene, proper handwashing is also suggested by the Food and Drug Administration:

- **Using** soap with warm running water (at least 100°F).
- **Vigorous** rubbing for 10–15 s
- **Rinsing** and drying hands with a clean disposable towel or a drying device.
- **Not** touching faucet handles after washing hands (e.g., turning off the faucet using a paper towel or motion sensor; Burusnukul and Broz 2013; Strohbehn et al. 2008).

If soap and water are not available, hand sanitizers are a convenient product that can reduce microbial pathogens from hand surfaces; however, hand sanitizers are not a complete replacement for proper handwashing. Thus, some viruses can resist the physiochemical inactivation and require vigorous friction during handwashing to be removed from the hands (Burusnukul and Broz 2013; Michaels 2004).

Thus, another suggestion is to ensure that signs are posted in common areas, which will reactivate the information that individuals may have already received in previous sanitation education or practices (Pragle et al. 2007) Also, it should be ensured that handwashing supplies and equipment are always available in convenient locations and working correctly. Further, it does not hurt to encourage and remind others to wash their hands more frequently (Burusnukul and Broz 2013).

Moreover, the CDC offers some important recommendations for when and how to wash one's hands. Hence, as mentioned before, keeping hands clean through improved hand hygiene is one of the most critical steps we can take to avoid getting sick and spreading germs to others. Many diseases and conditions are spread by not washing one's hands with soap and clean running water. Thus, if clean running water is not accessible, as is common in many parts of the world, use soap and available water, or utilize an alcohol-based hand sanitizer that contains at least 60% alcohol to clean your hands (CDC 2016).

When Should You Wash Your Hands?

Before, during, and after preparing food
Before eating food
Before and after caring for someone who is sick.
Before and after treatment with a cut or wound
After using the toilet
After changing diapers or cleaning up a child who has used the bathroom
After blowing your nose, coughing, or sneezing
After touching an animal, animal feed, or animal waste

After handling pet food or pet treatment **after** touching the garbage

How Should You Wash Your Hands?

Wet your hands with clean, running water (warm or cold), turn off the tap, and apply soap.

Lather your hands by rubbing them together with the soap. Be sure to lather the backs of your hands, between your fingers, and under your nails.

Scrub your hands for at least 20 seconds. Need a timer? Hum the "Happy Birthday" song from beginning to end twice.

Rinse your hands well under clean running water.

Dry your hands using a clean towel or air dry them.

What Should You do if You do not Have Soap and Clean Running Water?

Alcohol-based hand sanitizers containing at least 60% alcohol can quickly reduce the number of germs on the hands in some situations; however, sanitizers do not eliminate all types of germs and might not remove harmful chemicals (CDC 2016).

How Do You Use Hand Sanitizers?

Apply the product to the palm of one hand (read the label to learn the correct amount).

Rub your hands together.

Rub the product over all surface of your hands and fingers until your hands are dry (CDC 2016).

Indeed, it is essential to wash hands with soap and water or use hand sanitizer, which will reduce cross-contamination of germs.

However, while some authors mentioned the use of gloves a strategy to prevent disease transmission, recommendations regarding glove use are often segregated in other guidelines on isolation and personal protective equipment. Thus, in the context of patient care, it makes sense to think of glove use and hand hygiene as related elements of a comprehensive strategy to prevent transmission (Ellingson, Haas, Aiello, Kusek, Maragakis, Olmsted, and Yokoe 2014). In fact, handwashing is one of the most crucial steps of a comprehensive plan.

By all means, the authors of the studies presented in this paper offer some vital information, but more research is underway to prevent cross-contamination, such using hidden cameras to record handwashing behaviors and capture handwashing behaviors at various times, particularly in restrooms, restaurants, and patient rooms (Au, Suen, and Kwok 2010). Additionally, there must be further studies that focus on gender comparisons to see whether gender makes a difference, or age comparisons to see if such behaviors noted in adults can also be found in children (Au, Suen, and Kwok 2010).

Summary

Infection control is a broad topic, but it has various approaches and channels to focus the subject. Thus, the focus of this paper is on handwashing and the lack of handwashing in hospitals and various environments. Often, hands are dirty whether they appear dirty or not. Hands encounter many objects, and people who carry germs on their hands and body. Thus, the connection of dirty hands with another object or person has caused the transmission of bacteria to that object or person, which gives way to a chain of cross contamination that is not visible to the naked eye. Indeed, this is not a minor debate. Therefore, the war must be won to educate others about the transmission of disease so that there is a significant drop in cross-contamination. Bacteria lurk on most seemingly innocent surfaces awaiting our passing hands. *E. coli*, for instance, can survive on stainless steel for 60 days (Williams 1999).

Handwashing is the primary action that must be taken to kill germs. Many studies have shown that handwashing reduces infections. However, the message is lacking in some populations and cultures, even though it is essential knowledge that must be known to reduce cross-contamination and save lives. On the contrary, researchers who viewed behaviors and motivations as drivers to improve handwashing reported that having a positive belief and attitude toward handwashing provides a firm basis for a practical outcome (Burusnukul and Broz 2013).

Finally, addressing the rapid resistance of antibiotics to infections is simple. Start washing hands with soap and water often (antimicrobial soaps are unnecessary, and they may help spawn bacteria resistant to antibiotics). Hence, one knows that the adverse effects of handwashing are that frequent handwashing causes dry, cracked hands; however, lotions can be used to keep hands healthy and clean. As some say, in an age when antibiotics do not kill germs, soap and water will sure do the job, and do not forget the fingernails since eggs hide there (Williams 1999). Therefore, we should keep prioritizing education, awareness, reminders, and accountability to reduce cross-contamination and save lives.

Thus, to be sure you do not give up while washing, sing "Twinkle, Twinkle, Little Star" (Williams 1999).

REFERENCES

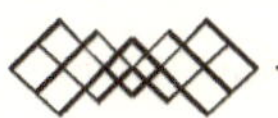

Au, W. H., Suen, L. K. P., and Kwok, Y. L. 2010. "Handwashing Programmed in Kindergarten: A Pilot Study." 110(1), 5–16. https://search. proquest.com/pqrlprintviewfile?accountid=41759.

Australian Government Department of Health. 2010. "8 Food Poisoning and contaminations." http://www.health.gov.au/internet/publications/publishing.nsf/Content/ohp-enhealth-manual-atsi-cnt-l-ohp-enhealth-manual-atsi-cnt-l-ch3-ohpen-health-manual-atsi-cnt-l-ch3.8.

Bawaba, A. 2014. "The United States: Dow Announces an Affiliation with the Global Public-Private Partnership for Handwashing with Soap." https://search.proquest.com/pqrl/docview/16422712750/4cc9aflf28084659pq/15?accoun-tid=41759.

Bischoff, W. E., Rynolds, T. M., Sessler, C. N., Edmond, M. B., and Wenzzel, R. P. 2000. "Handwashing Compliance by Health Care Workers: The Impact of Introducing an Accessible, Alcohol-Based Hand Antiseptic." *Archives of Internal Medicine* 160(7), 1017–21. https://search.proquest.com/pqrl/ printviewfile?accountid?accountid-41759.

Bjerke, N. B. 2004. "The Evolution: Handwashing to Hand Hygiene Guidance." *Critical Care Nursing Quarterly* 27(3), 295–307. https://search.proquest.com/pqrl/ printviewfile?accountid =41759.

Boshell, P. 2016. "Hand Hygiene at Home and School." https://infectioncontrol.tips/2016/08/19/hand-hygiene-home-school/.

Boyce and Pitt, D. 2002. "Guideline for and Hygiene in Health-Care Settings." https://www.cdc.gov/mmwr/preview/mmwrhtml/rr5116al.htm.

Burusnukul, P., and Broz, C. C. 2013. "Drivers and Motivators in Consumer Handwashing Behavior." 43(6), 596–604. https://doi:10.1108/NFS-01-2013-0010.

Center for Disease Control and Prevention. 2016. "Improving Adherence to Hand Hygiene Practice: A Multidisciplinary Approach." https://wwwnc.cdc.gov/ article /7/2/70-0234_article.

Center for Disease Control and Prevention. 2016. "When and How to Wash Your Hands." https://www.cdc.gov/handwashing/when-how-handwashing.html.

Center for Disease Control and Prevention. 2018. "HAI Data and Statistics." https://www.cdc.gov/hai/surveillance/index.html.

Center for Disease Control and Prevention. 2020. "Global Handwashing Day." cdc.gov/handwashing/index.html.

Davis, R. 2015. "The Doctor Who Championed Handwashing and Briefly Saved Lives." https://www.npr.org/sections/health-shots/2015/01/12/375663920/the-doctor-who-championed-hand-washing-and-saved-women-s-lives.

Ellingson, K., Haas, J. P., Aiello, E., Kysek, L., Maragakis, L. L., Olmssted, R. N., and Yokoe, D. S. 2014. "Strategies to Prevent Healthcare-Associated Infections through Hand Hygiene." https://doi:10.1086/677145.

Federal Register/Finf; Washington. 2010. "Infectious Diseases." 75(087), 24835. https://search.proquest.com/pqr// printview file?accountid=41759.

Gale Encyclopedia. 2006. "Food Poisoning." https://www. encyclopedia. com/medicine/diseases-and-condition/pathology/food poisoning.

Gale Encyclopedia. 2008. "Infection Control." https://medical-dictionary.thefreedictionary.com/infection+control.

Garba, L., Dayyab, F. M., Habib, Z. G., Tiamiyu, A. B., Abubakar, S., Mijinyawa, M. S., and Habib, A. G. 2016. "Knowledge and Practices of Infection Control among Healthcare

Workers in a Tertiary Referral Center in North-Western Nigeria." *Annals of African Medicine* 15(1), 34–40. https://doi:10.4103/1596-3519.161724.

Gibson, B. E., and Markovic. 2015. "Immediate and Maintenance Effects of the Intervention on Handwashing Compliance in Healthcare Workers." http://ideawxchange.uakron.edu/honors_research_projects.

Girou, E. Loyeau, S., Legrand, P. Oppein, F., and Brun-Buisson, C. 2002. "Efficacy of Hand Rubbing with an AlcoholBased Solution versus Standard Handwashing with Antiseptic Soap: Randomized Clinical Trial." www.bmj.com/ content/325/7360/362.

Hingley, A. 1997. "Focus on Food Safety." United Food and Drug Administration. http://www.thebody.com/content/art13864.html.

Hugonnet, S., Perneger, T. V., and Pittet, D. 2002. "Alcohol-Based Hand Rub Improves Compliance with Hand Hygiene in Intensive Care Units." 162(9), 1037–43. https://search.proquest.com/ pqrl/printviewfile?accountid=41759.

Larson, E. L., Cloonan, E., Sandra, S., and Parides, M. 2000. "An Organizational Climate Intervention Associated with Increased Handwashing and Decreased Nosocomial Infections." 26(1), 14. https://search.proquest.com/ docview/195226007?accountid=41759.

London. 2014. "United States: Dow Announces an Affiliation with the Global Public-Private Partnership for Handwashing with Soap."

Lusk, M. L. 1996. For Good or Ill, the Great Unwashed Are Making a Comeback." *Nation's Restaurant News* 30(29), 26. https://search.proquest.com/docview/229264428?accountid=41759.

Mathur, P. 2011. "Hand Hygiene: Back to the Basics of Infection Control." *Indian Journal of Medical Research*. 134(5), 611–20. Retrieved from https://doi:10.4103/0971-5916.90985.

Med, S. A. 2007. "A Brief History of Infection Control—Past and Present." 97 (11 pt. 3), 1161–4. https://www.ncbi.nim.nih.gov/ pubmed/18250929.

Miller, J. T., Rahimi, S., and Lee, M. 2005. "History of Infection Control and Its Contributions to the Development and Success of Brain Tumor Operations." 18(4). https://www.ncbl.nlm.nih.gov/ pubmed/15844867.

Minnesota Department of Health. 2017. "Five Common Ways Germs Are Spread." (14) 25. http://www.health.state.mn.us/handhygiene/why/5ways.html.

Mosby's Medical Dictionary. 2009. "Bacteria." https://medical-dictionary.thefreedictionary.com/bacteria.

Mosby's Medical Dictionary. 2012. "Cross Contamination." https://medical-dictionary.thefreedictionary.com/cross contamination.

Pragle, A. S., and Harding, A. K. 2007. "Food Workers' Perspectives on Handwashing Behaviors and Barriers in the Restaurant Environment." *JournalofEnvironmentalHealth*69(10),27.https://search.proquest.com/docview/219709048?accountid=41759.

Pyrek, K. M. 2004. "Infection Control Today—03/2004: Handwashing and Cross contamination." http://www.infectioncontroltoday.com/articles/2004/03/infection-control-today-03-2004-handwashing-and-c.aspx.

Sender, R., Fuchs, S., and Milo, R. 2016. "Are We Really Vastly Outnumbered? Revisiting the Ratio of Bacterial to Host Cells in Humans." http://dx.doi.org/10.1016/j.cell.2016.01.013.

Teare, L., Cookson, B., French, G., and Jenner, E. 2000. "Handwashing—Myth or Magic?" *Health and Hygiene* 21(2), 66. https://search. proquest.com/docview/205501240?accountid=41759.

The Stateman, New Delhi. 2002. "Health: Don't Catch It If You Can." https://search.proquest.com/pqrl/printviewfile?accountid=41759.

Turkoski, B. B. 2005. "Fighting Infection an Ongoing Challenge." Part 1: *Orthopedic Nursing* 24(1), 40. https://www.ncbinim.nih.goo/pubmed/15722973.

Williams III, G. 1999. "The Biology of... Handwashing." http://discovermagazine.com/1999/dec.feathand.

World Health Organization.2013. "Evidence of hand hygiene to reduce transmission and infections by multidrug resistant organisms in health-care settings." www.who.int

World Health Organization. 2020. "Disease(COVID-19) Dashboard". https://covid19.who.int.

Yakob, E. L., Lamaro, T., and Henok, A. 2015. "Knowledge, Attitude, and Practice towards Infection Control Measures among Mizana-Man General Hospital Workers." *South West Ethiopia: Journal of Community Medicine & Health Education* 5(370). Retrieved from https://doi: 10.4172/21610711.1000370.

APPENDIX A

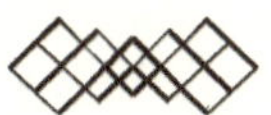

1.1 Ways food can become contaminated through incorrect food handling.

Food can become contaminated with disease-causing bacteria anywhere the food is handled or stored. These places include the following:

- In a factory where it is processed for sale
- In a truck in which it is taken from the factory to the shop
- In a shop
- In a food outlet such as a school canteen or take-away shop
- between the shop and home
- At home

Most food has to be prepared in some way before it is eaten. During this preparation, the food is handled by people. There are many ways in which unhygienic practices can cause food poisoning bacteria to be deposited on food while it is being handled. Some examples are as follows:

- Leaving food uncovered. Pets, flies, cockroaches, and other insects carry germs, including food poisoning bacteria, which contaminate the food
- Touching parts of the body while handling food While preparing food, a food handler might scratch a pimple, touch a sore, push back hair, scratch an ear, or rub or pick the nose. Every one of these activities contaminates the fingers

with bacteria. If the person's hands are not washed before handling food again, these bacteria will be passed to the food. **Figure A.1

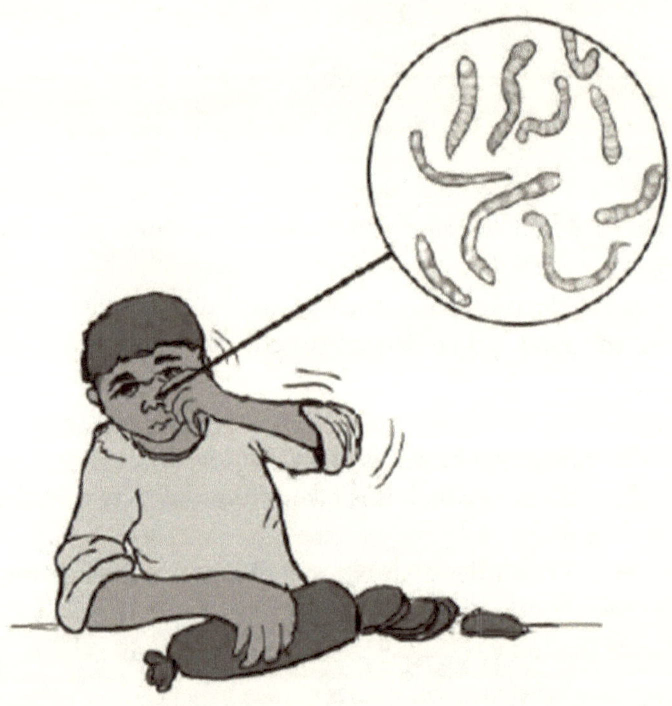

**Figure 1.3: Rubbing the nose while preparing food
helps spread germs.

- Sneezing or coughing near food. If a food handler, or anyone else, sneezes or coughs near uncovered food, then the food almost will certainly be sprayed with bacteria-laden droplets.

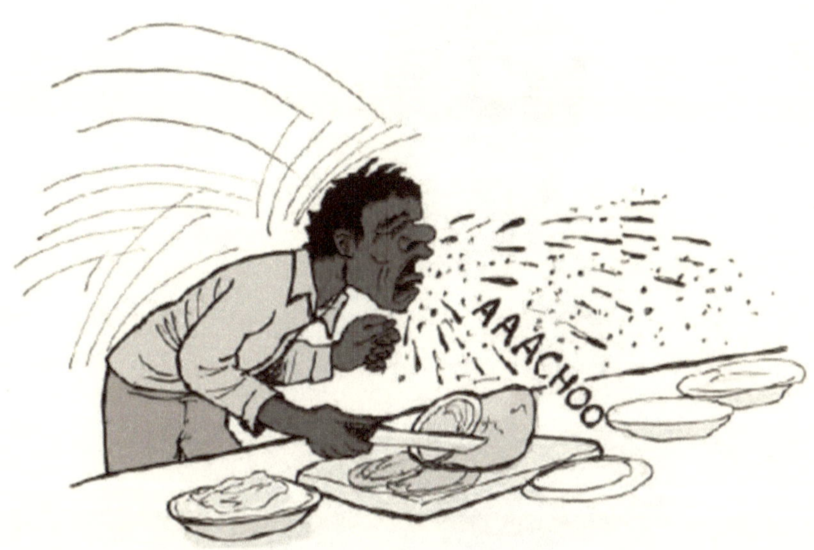

**Figure A.2: Sneezing over food spreads germs.

- Licking fingers while handling food human saliva carries staphylococcus bacteria and licking the fingers could result in the bacteria being passed to the food.

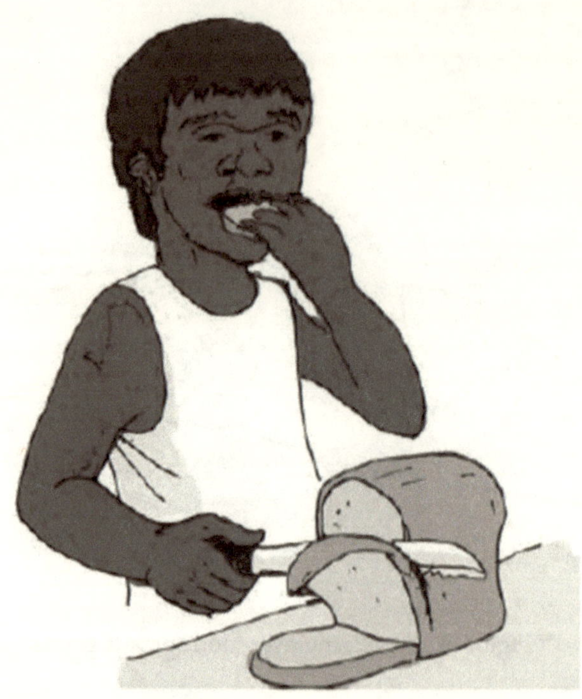

**Figure A.3: Licking fingers while handling food spreads germs

- Not washing hands after going to the toilet during food handling. If a person goes to the toilet during food handling activities and does not wash his/her hands afterwards, food poisoning bacteria may be passed onto the food.

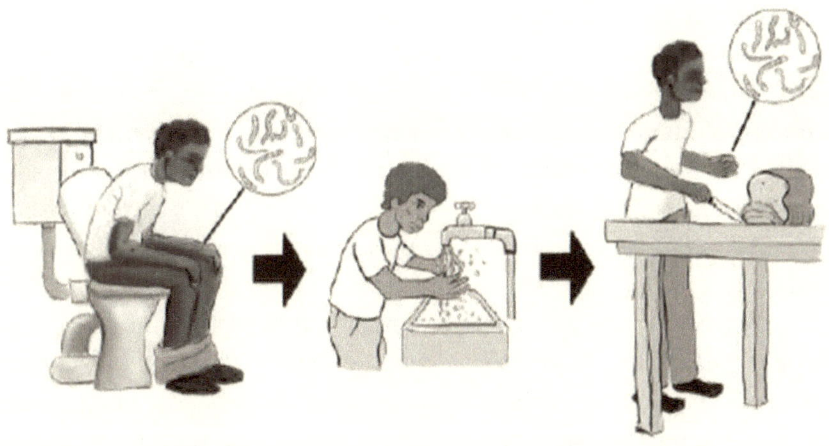

**Figure A.4: Washing hands after going to the
toilet helps stop the spread of germs.

- Poor handling of high-risk foods. High-risk foods are those who generally need refrigeration and have a high moisture content. Poor handling of high-risk foods is a common cause of food poisoning. High-risk foods include the following:

  - chicken, duck, and other poultry
  - fish and shellfish
  - raw meat products
  - dairy products (milk, cheese, and cream)
  - unpasteurized cow or goat milk
  - eggs and egg products
  - gravies

Cross-contamination. Certain foods will always contain some bacteria. Poor handling of these foods may result in **cross-contamination**. Cross-contamination is the passing of bacteria from contaminated food to uncontaminated food. Cross-contamination can occur when storing or handling food.

An example of cross-contamination during storage is:

High-risk food, such as raw chicken thawing in a refrigerator, is placed in contact with cooked meat. The bacteria from the raw chicken contaminate the cooked meat. Since the cooked meat is not heated again before eating, the bacteria from the chicken pass to the person who eats the meat.

An example of cross-contamination during handling is as follows:

Before cooking a fish that is contaminated with Salmonella bacteria, a person uses a knife and cutting board to cut it up. Bacteria from the fish will be left on the knife and cutting board. The person slices cooked ham using the same knife and board without washing them first. The bacteria were transferred to the ham.

**Department of Health (2010) Retrieved from https://www.health. gov. au/internet/publications/publishing.nsf/Content/ohp-enhealth-manual-atsi-cnt-l-ohp-enhealth-manual-atsi-cnt-l-ch3-ohpen-health-manual-atsi-cnt-l-ch3.8

DEFINITIONS

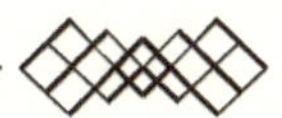

1. Puerperal fever (pathology) is a systemic bacterial infection of the endometrium characterized by fever, rapid heartbeat, uterine tenderness, and malodorous discharge, mainly occurring in women after childbirth, usually as a result of unsterile obstetric procedures. Puerperal fever. (n.d.). *Dictionary.com*, Unabridged. Retrieved from the Dictionary. com.
2. Antibiotic (Greek *anti* "against," *bios* "life") refers to substances produced by some microorganisms to suppress the growth of other microorganisms (Turkoski 2005).

APPENDIX B

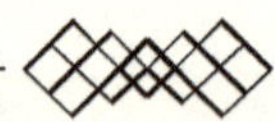

Don't Forget to Wash

This simple poster (available in two color options) shows six simple steps to washing hands.

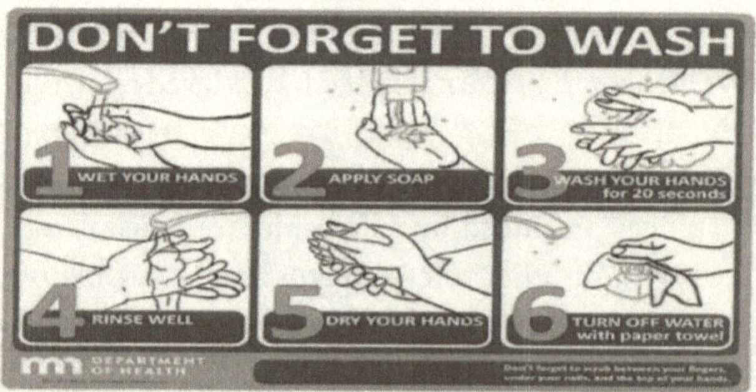

Download a print version:
Don't Forget to Wash (PDF)
(http://www.health.state.mn.us/handhygiene/wash/dontforget.pdf)

Don't Forget to Wash

1. Wet your hands
2. Apply soap
3. Wash your hands for 20 seconds

5. Dry your hands
6. Turn off water with a paper towel

Also available in color:

(http://www.health.state.mn.us/handhygiene/wash/dontforgetc.pdf)

Don't Forget to Wash (color) (PDF)
(http://www.health.state.mn.us/handhygiene/wash/dontforgetc.pdf)

Updated Friday, 20-Oct-2017 12:23:42 CDT

APPENDIX C

Certificate of Completion

The National Institutes of Health (NIH) Office of Extramural Research certifies that Teresa Mabry successfully completed the NIH Web-based training course "Protecting Human Research Participants."

Date of Completion: 04/09/2018

Certification Number: 2630965

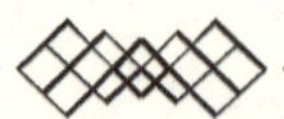

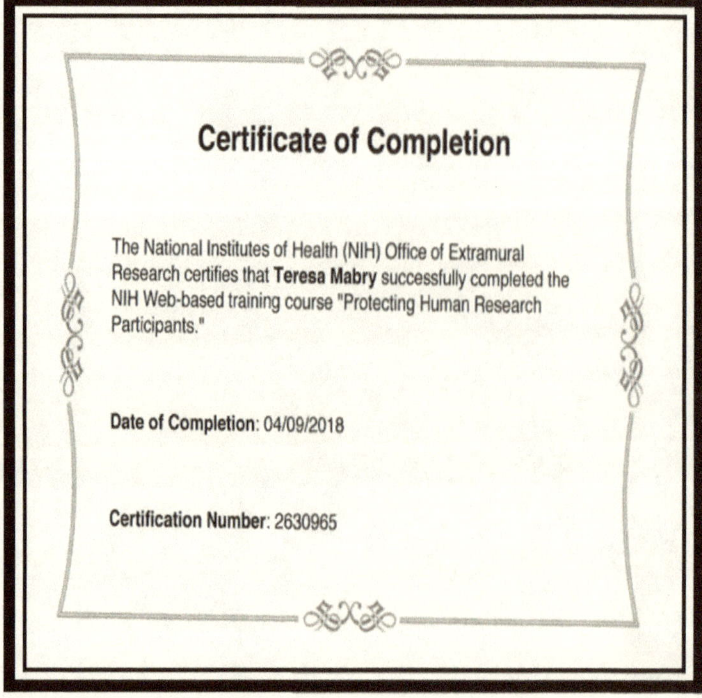

*Jesus is watching everywhere so
Wash your hands everywhere because
Jesus and germs are everywhere.*

About the Author

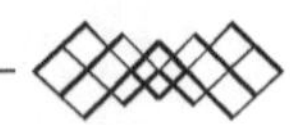

Teresa Mabry currently resides in Emporia, Virginia, with her husband and three poodles. She graduated with an associate degree in applied science. She worked in the medical industry in acute and chronic facilities as a respiratory therapist for fifteen years. During this time, she noticed the significant need for people to wash their hands. Teresa's parents have always enforced handwashing in the home growing up; neither did the parents allow family members or anyone to participate in food preparations or eat unless hands were washed. The importance of handwashing and cleanliness was carried over into adulthood for Teresa and her family. The discipline taught on purity has made a difference in being infected and transmitting a bacterium.

The enjoyment of being amongst people and keeping people healthy has led her return to school for a bachelor's degree in respiratory care management, then the master's degree in healthcare administration. The master's degree program is where Teresa was given the opportunity to author a book and express in writing the critical need to wash the hands. A date that has coincided with keeping persons safe and healthy, October 15. The National Global Handwashing Day. The same date as the author's birthday was established on October 15, 2008 by the Global Handwashing Partnership.

www.ingramcontent.com/pod-product-compliance
Lightning Source LLC
Chambersburg PA
CBHW031146250726
48655CB00002B/867